SILENT WAR

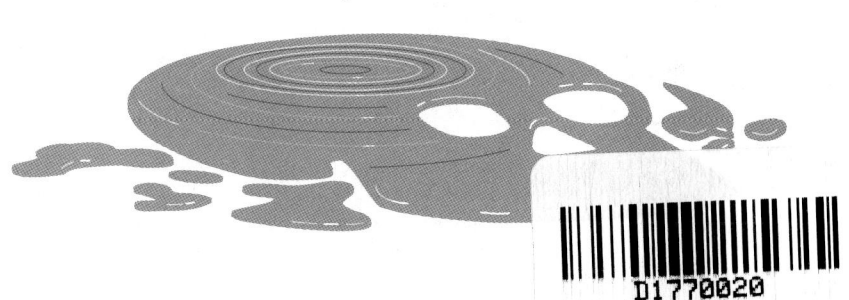

INFECTION CONTROL FOR LAW ENFORCEMENT

STUDENT TEXTBOOK

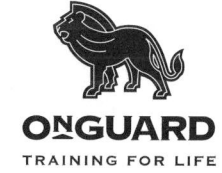

ON**GUARD**
TRAINING FOR LIFE

Infection control and emergency response are not exact sciences, and they involve many unknown variables. The course *Silent War: Infection Control for Law Enforcement* is not intended to provide all the training necessary for safe infection control procedures and emergency response. OnGUARD will not be responsible for any misunderstanding or misapplication of the information presented in this program. In addition, OnGUARD will not be liable for any injury or death resulting from the application of information presented in this course.

Project Manager: Pam Glossi
Editor: Susan Peterson
Illustrations: Ken Keegan
Graphics: Jeff Northway
Cover Design: Wilson-Johnson Creative

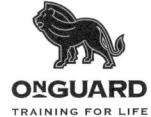

© 1993, 1996 by OnGUARD, Inc.
Fort Collins, Colorado

All rights reserved. No part of this program may be reproduced in any form or by any means. Unless specific written permission is obtained from OnGUARD, it is expressly prohibited to:

- Copy or duplicate the videotapes or instructional materials for any reason.
- Rent or lend this training program or charge fees for viewing.
- Copy the videotapes for archive purposes. Duplicate or replacement copies are available at substantially reduced costs through OnGUARD.
- Transmit this video program in whole or in part by broadcast, cable, or satellite. If you wish to transmit this program via cable broadcast or satellite within your own organization, please call OnGUARD for fee schedule information.

This video training program was created at the lowest possible cost to you, while maintaining the highest standards of quality and content. Please respect our mutual best interests and refrain from duplicating this program. If you are aware of a copyright violation, call OnGUARD at 1-800-544-3473 (U.S. and Canada).

ISBN 1-56916-710-9
Printed in the United States of America

March 1996

Introduction

    Course Instructors ix
    Acknowledgements xiii

Tape 1:
Understanding Contagious Diseases

Session 1:
Why Is Infection Control Necessary? ... 1

OBJECTIVE: Explain why you as a law enforcement officer should be trained in preventing the spread of communicable diseases 2

    Communicable Diseases Are on the Rise 3
    Officers Face Increased Exposure Risk 7
    Officers Have a Duty to Protect Themselves
        and Others 10
    Developing Legal Issues 12

    SUMMARY 14

Session 2:
Understanding the Silent Assailant 17

OBJECTIVE: State how communicable diseases are spread 18

    Infectious Agent 20
    Mode of Transmission 21
    Portal of Entry 24
    Receiving Host 25
    Body Substance Isolation 26

OBJECTIVE: Identify general precautions you
can take to protect yourself from contracting a
communicable disease 30

    Get Hepatitis B Vaccination
        and TB Screening 31
    Use Personal Protective Equipment 32
    Take Precautions After Exposure 34
    Stay Healthy 35

SUMMARY 35

Tape 2:
Reducing Your Risk

Session 3:
The Balancing Act 39

OBJECTIVE: Describe the personal decontamination procedures you should follow if you've been
exposed to blood or other body fluids that might
be infectious 41

    Remove Contaminated Clothing 42
    Wash Hands and Skin 43
    Cleanse Eyes, Nose, and Mouth 44

OBJECTIVE: Identify infection control concerns
you should have when entering a crime scene . . 45

    Protect Yourself 46
    Don't Spread Body Fluids 46
    Don't Expose Others 47

OBJECTIVE: Given a specific situation, determine whether personal protective equipment
should be used and, if so, what type 48

    Wear Gloves 49
    Use Other PPE 51
    Cover Damaged Skin 52

OBJECTIVE: Identify proper procedures for
handling needles and sharp evidence 53

    Handle Needles Safely 53
    Use a Puncture Resistant Container 54

OBJECTIVE: Describe the precautions you
should follow when handling a dead body 56

    Don't Touch 56
    Use BSI Procedures 57

OBJECTIVE: List the types of personal protective
equipment you should use when giving first aid
to a person 59

    Put on Gloves 59
    Use an Airway Device 61

SUMMARY 61

Session 4:
Arrests, Searches, Vehicle Decon **63**

OBJECTIVE: Describe the risk of contracting a
communicable disease when arresting a suspect,
and state the precautions you should take to
minimize the possibility of disease transmission . 65

    Spitting 65
    Biting 66
    Patdowns 67

OBJECTIVE: Identify precautions you should
take when conducting a vehicle search to
minimize the risk of exposure to a communicable
disease 69

    Use PPE 70
    Look Before Reaching 70

OBJECTIVE: Outline proper procedures for
decontaminating a vehicle 72

    Use PPE 72

Soak Up Spills	73
Preclean	73
Disinfect	74
Air Dry	74
SUMMARY	75

Tape 3:
Post-Incident Procedures

Session 5:
Collecting Evidence 77

OBJECTIVE: Outline precautions you should take while investigating a "cold" crime scene	78
Wear Gloves	79
Don't Put Things in Your Mouth	79
OBJECTIVE: List procedures you should follow when collecting evidence	80
Wear Other PPE	81
Minimize Splashing	82
Use Tape, Not Staples	83
Use Tweezers for Glass	83
Use Warning Labels	84
Handle Collection Tools Properly	85
OBJECTIVE: Summarize the steps you should follow to decontaminate yourself and your equipment after collecting evidence	86
Remove PPE	87
Remove and Clean Contaminated Clothing	88
Wash Hands and Skin	88
Decontaminate Nondisposable Items	89
SUMMARY	89

Session 6:
Bookings and Legal Issues 91

OBJECTIVE: Identify precautions you should take when fingerprinting and searching a prisoner to guard against exposure to a communicable disease 92

    Wear Gloves 93
    Have Prisoners Empty Pockets 94
    Wear Face/Eye Protection for Coughing 95

OBJECTIVE: State the procedures you should follow in cleaning a cell so there will be minimal risk of exposure to a communicable disease 96

    Wear PPE 97
    Decontaminate Cell 97
    Dispose of or Decontaminate
        Cleaning Materials 98
    Decontaminate Yourself 99

OBJECTIVE: Summarize the major legal issues relating to infection control that law enforcement agencies need to address 100

    No Discrimination 102
    OSHA and CDC 102
    Job Discrimination 104
    Confidentiality 106
    Ryan White Act 109
    Workers' Compensation 110
    Training 110
    Other Prison Issues 112
    A Step Further 113

  SUMMARY 115

Appendix 119

    Exposure Control Guidelines for Common
        Communicable Diseases 120

Course Instructors

John Anderson

Sgt. John Anderson began his law enforcement career in 1972. His primary areas of expertise are in the fields of criminal investigations and police training. He is a former homicide investigator and has also been a staff instructor at the Police Training Academy in Colorado Springs, Colorado. He is currently assigned to the Office of Professional Standards for the Colorado Springs Police Department.

Tom Bay

Lt. Tom Bay is currently serving in the Training Section of the Arapahoe County Sheriff's Office in Littleton, Colorado. He also has 10 years of experience with the Arapahoe County Detention Center.

Roger Burchett

Capt. Roger Burchett has been a member of the Jefferson County Sheriff's Department in Golden, Colorado since 1966. He is presently the Division Commander in the Department's Informational Services Division. He has extensive training and experience in the fields of polygraph and investigative hypnosis. He has also served as an administrator in several other Divisions of the Department, including three years as Commander of the Department's Investigation Section.

Tim Dunning

Lt. Tim Dunning has served with the Police Department in Omaha, Nebraska since 1973. He is currently the Commander for the Omaha Police Training Section. Other assignments have included the Gang Unit, the Narcotics Unit, and the Organized Crime Unit. Lt. Dunning has conducted over 100 public presentations and has been a guest lecturer and instructor for numerous classes. He is a graduate of the FBI National Academy.

Twink Gorgen

Twink Gorgen has served as a staff nurse and paramedic instructor since 1974. She is presently the paramedic nurse coordinator and a field supervisor for the EMS Division of the Fire Department in Omaha, Nebraska. She has taught numerous courses, has given seminars at several national conferences, and has conducted state and local workshops. She has written several articles and is a contributing author for three textbooks for paramedics.

Steve Holl

Lt. Steve Holl joined the Arlington County Police Department in Arlington, Virginia in 1973. He currently commands the Staff Support Section and is the Infection Control Officer for the Department. He has also served as Commander of the Special Operations Section and as Commander of the SWAT Team and Hostage Negotiation Team. He is a graduate of the FBI National Academy.

Ron Leavell

Ron Leavell is presently serving as Health Services Administrator for the Arapahoe County Detention Center in Englewood, Colorado. A retired Army Nurse Corps officer, Mr. Leavell has 30 years of nursing experience, including Clinic Administrator/Infection Control Officer.

Jim Lynch

Capt. Jim Lynch is an 18 year veteran of the Arlington County Fire Department in Arlington, Virginia. He is presently the EMS Training Coordinator and also coordinates the Emergency Response Team Medical Support. He has conducted training programs for local and federal law enforcement agencies, for the Virginia State Division of EMS on satellite and video programs, and for the State EMS Symposium.

Carol Shanaberger

The late Carol Shanaberger had a 15 year history as an attorney at law. Concurrent with her legal practice, she served as an EMT/paramedic for 12 years. The emphasis of Ms. Shanaberger's legal practice was on consulting services regarding EMS medical and legal issues. She also served as an investigator for the Colorado Department of Regulatory Agencies and as an EMS liaison for the Colorado Board of Medical Examiners. She contributed to several books and wrote a monthly column for the *Journal of Emergency Medical Services* on legal aspects of prehospital services. She conducted dozens of seminars nationwide on EMS legal issues.

Acknowledgements

Many people were involved in the production of this training program. We want to acknowledge the instructors we worked with, who faithfully offered their talents, experience, and professional guidance in spite of their own demanding schedules:

Sgt. John Anderson, Colorado Springs, CO
Lt. Tom Bay, Arapahoe County, CO
Capt. Roger Burchett, Jefferson County, CO
Lt. Tim Dunning, Omaha, NE
Twink Gorgen, Omaha, NE
Lt. Steve Holl, Arlington County, VA
Ron Leavell, Arapahoe County, CO
Capt. Jim Lynch, Arlington County, VA
Chief Dennis Rubin, Chesterfield, VA
Carol Shanaberger, Lakewood, CO

We are also grateful to our technical reviewers, who shared their suggestions as the textbook took shape:

Sgt. John Anderson, Colorado Springs, CO
Carl Bart, Pasadena, MD
Lt. Tom Bay, Arapahoe County, CO
Sgt. Michael Black, Dallas, TX
Capt. Roger Burchett, Jefferson County, CO
Sgt. Thomas Curran, Wallingford, CT
Chief Douglas Dortenzio, Wallingford, CT
Lt. Tim Dunning, Omaha, NE
Sgt. Chris Ellis, San Diego, CA
Timothy Erickson, St. Paul, MN
Lt. Steve Holl, Arlington County, VA
Capt. Jim Lynch, Arlington County, VA
Steve Otto, Dallas, TX
Sgt. Ken Petersen, Arvada, CO
Carol Shanaberger, Lakewood, CO
Earl M. Sweeney, Concord, NH
Sgt. Steve Ward, Colorado Springs, CO

Special thanks to members of the OnGUARD team: Mark Sprenger, president of OnGUARD, for his vision and initiative; Joe Varela, director of program development, for his tireless management and oversight of the project; Pam Glossi, project manager, for her efforts in coordinating, editing, and scheduling; Bob Bing, for developing the curriculum; Susan Peterson, for writing, editing, and formatting the text; Jeff Northway, for designing the graphics; and Dixie McKeehan, for providing clerical support. We also acknowledge Ken Keegan, who supplied the cartoons.

This infection control program could not have been completed without all of these participants. Our thanks to everyone.

SESSION 1
Why Is Infection Control Necessary?

As a law enforcement officer, you're at risk of exposure to communicable diseases. No matter what your duties—whether you're rendering first aid, arresting a suspect, booking a prisoner, controlling an assailant, processing a crime scene, investigating a traffic accident, or responding to a domestic dispute—you have the potential of coming in contact with body fluids, contaminated needles, and airborne particles that may be infectious. If you work in a correctional institution, you routinely deal with individuals whose past or present behaviors place them at high risk of developing diseases such as AIDS and hepatitis B. In some prisons, tuberculosis, another communicable disease, infects up to 50% of inmates.[1]

> **Officers are at risk of exposure to communicable diseases.**

Communicable diseases (also known as contagious diseases) can be thought of as silent assailants. They don't shout or brandish guns, but they can be deadly in their assaults. To avoid becoming infected with a communicable disease, you need to know how such diseases are transmitted and how to protect your own health and the health of the people you serve. Training in these areas is essential. After reading this session and viewing the accompanying videotape, you should be able to achieve the following objective:

> **OBJECTIVE: Explain why you as a law enforcement officer should be trained in preventing the spread of communicable diseases.**

Key Points

1. *Communicable diseases are on the rise.* These diseases include not only **HIV/AIDS,** but also **hepatitis B, tuberculosis,** and other diseases.

2. As a police officer, you face an *increased risk of being exposed* to or becoming infected with a communicable disease on the job.

3. You have a *duty to protect* yourself, your family and loved ones, your coworkers, the people you deal with, and the community you serve from communicable diseases.

4. There are *developing legal concerns* regarding citizens' civil rights in areas such as confidentiality of communicable disease status and discrimination based on disease status.

© 1996 OnGUARD, Inc.

Communicable Diseases Are on the Rise

As a peace officer, you have a very challenging, yet unpredictable and stressful job. You never know what you might run into during a shift. You must be ready to respond to any emergency, whether it is participating in a drug bust, quieting a disturbance in a jail, arresting a suspect, rendering first aid to a traffic accident victim, or performing any of a multitude of other tasks. As if these situations weren't stressful enough, you're expected to carry out your duties under any and all weather and lighting conditions. To make matters worse, an increasing number of the people you have to deal with may have HIV or some other disease, and

> **Officers must find the right balance between performing their duties and protecting themselves.**

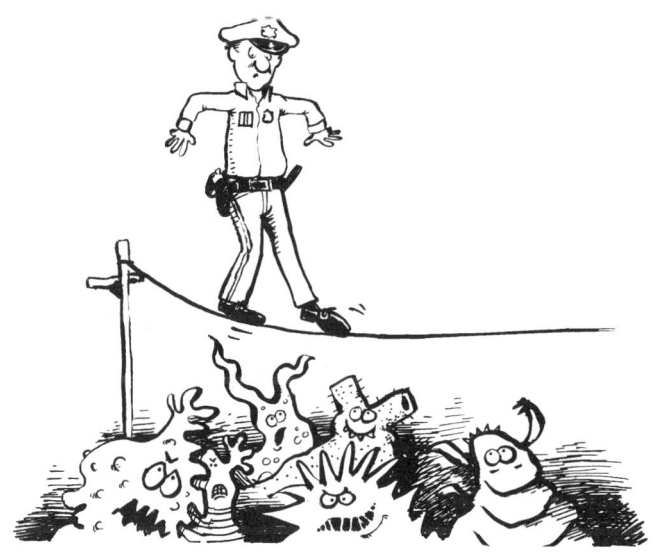

Find the Right Balance

© 1996 OnGUARD, Inc.

Silent War

you can't help but be concerned about your own health and safety. You find you have to weigh the things you do as you respond to each emergency call against a personal obligation to protect yourself from harm. Finding the right balance is a challenge you face every day. Understanding communicable diseases can help make that challenge easier.

A **communicable disease** is a disease that can be transmitted from one person to another through direct or indirect contact. Acquired Immune Deficiency Syndrome (AIDS) is an example of a communicable disease that has received much attention in recent years because of its rapid spread worldwide and devastating fatality rate. In 1981, there were 309 cases of AIDS reported in the United States. Five years later the cumulative total had risen to 30,139 cases. By the end of June 1995, a total of 476,899 cases

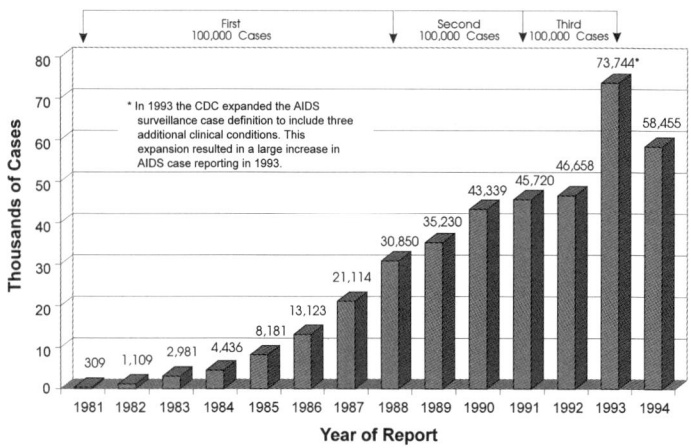

Source: Centers for Disease Control and Prevention

Figure 1-1. The Rise of AIDS in the United States

© 1996 OnGUARD, Inc.

had been reported in the United States, of which 295,473 had died.[2] The World Health Organization estimates that as of January 3, 1995, 18 million adults and 1.5 million children worldwide have been infected with human immunodeficiency virus (HIV), the virus that causes AIDS. The worldwide total is projected to be 30-40 million by 2000.

Hepatitis B is another communicable disease. It is less well known than AIDS but can be just as serious. The hepatitis B virus is spread primarily through sexual transmission and exposure to infected blood. An estimated 300,000 people in the United States are infected by the virus each year. Approximately 4,000 Americans die each year from cirrhosis of the liver caused by hepatitis B, and another 800 die each year from primary liver cancer caused by hepatitis B.[3] First responders such as law enforcement officers, firefighters, and emergency medical service (EMS) personnel are particularly at risk for contracting hepatitis B because their jobs frequently involve exposure to blood. Other types of hepatitis (hepatitis A, C, D, and E) also present a risk to emergency personnel. These types are summarized in the appendix.

> **Officers are at risk for contracting hepatitis B because their jobs involve exposure to blood.**

Tuberculosis (TB) is also on the rise. The number of reported cases of TB in the United States steadily dropped from 84,304 patients in 1953 to 22,255 in 1984. However, since 1984, this long-term decline has stopped. Over the last few years an average of 25,000 TB cases have been reported annually in the United States. Nearly 70% of the cases in recent years have occurred among racial and ethnic minorities.[4]

The reversal in the downward trend of tuberculosis is believed to be caused by the following factors:

> **Tuberculosis is a major problem in prisons and among the poor and homeless.**

- the growing homeless and medically underserved low income populations
- an increasing number of people living in close settings, such as the elderly in nursing homes and inmates in correctional facilities
- the influx of people from countries where the disease appears in large numbers
- the HIV epidemic (many HIV patients are also infected with TB)
- the increase in alcoholism and drug abuse
- the increase in the occurrence of drug resistant strains of tuberculosis[5]

The incidence of measles has also increased in recent years. In the late 1980s and early 1990s there was more than a five-fold increase in the number of cases reported annually in the United States. Measles and several other diseases were once considered nearly eradicated, but recent outbreaks have reversed the trend. These childhood diseases, which also include whooping cough, diphtheria, mumps, chicken pox, and polio, should not be dismissed lightly. They can have serious complications for adults.

Other communicable diseases that you should be aware of include meningitis, herpes viruses, and influenza. A chart listing the major communicable diseases, their methods of transmission, the relative risk for police officers, recommended precautions to take, and procedures to follow in the event of exposure is included in the appendix.

Officers Face Increased Exposure Risk

Because of the increasing prevalence of communicable diseases in the general population, as a peace officer you run a greater risk of exposure while on duty. An *exposure* is defined as direct contact of an infectious agent such as a body fluid, droplet, or aerosol with an open wound, area of broken skin, or mucous membrane of the eyes, nose, or mouth, or piercing the skin with a contaminated sharp instrument.

Don't think you'll escape exposure just because you work in a small community. Intravenous (IV) drug users in big cities aren't the only people who can place you at risk. On the contrary, the risk of communicable disease exposure in suburban communities and among the heterosexual population has increased **significantly** in the last few years. No matter where you work, you face an increased exposure risk.

> **There is a significant risk of exposure in suburban communities and among heterosexuals.**

In the law enforcement profession, depending on the particular disease, exposures can occur in many ways. To name a few:

- through cuts and puncture wounds while you're conducting searches and patdowns
- through saliva, respiratory secretions, and vomit while you're administering CPR or first aid
- through biting and spitting by combative offenders
- through contact with urine or feces
- through proximity to someone who's coughing
- through contact with body fluids on a corpse

© 1996 OnGUARD, Inc.

- through contact with body fluids during scene searches, when no one is around

If you encounter these situations frequently, you face a greater probability of being exposed to a communicable disease. Because **any** exposure incident can lead to infection, training in preventing the spread of communicable diseases is vital.

Another reason you and your fellow officers face an increased exposure risk is that you often must deal with individuals whose past or present behaviors place them at high risk of being infected with a communicable disease. IV drug users, for example, are a high risk group for HIV. Most of the behaviors that increase the risk of HIV infection also increase the risk of contracting hepatitis B, tuberculosis, and other communicable diseases. Figure 1-2 presents a summary of high risk behaviors for some of the major communicable diseases.

> **Officers often must deal with people who are at high risk of being infected with communicable diseases.**

High Risk Behaviors for Common Communicable Diseases

HIV Infection

- ✓ Sharing IV needles
- ✓ Receiving multiple blood or blood product transfusions
- ✓ Unprotected sex with infected persons
- ✓ Infants born to HIV infected mothers

Hepatitis B

- ✓ Sharing IV needles
- ✓ Improper waste disposal
- ✓ Poor personal hygiene
- ✓ Unprotected sex with infected persons

Tuberculosis

- ✓ Residing in close quarters with infected persons
- ✓ Residing in unsanitary conditions
- ✓ Exposing a person whose immune system has been weakened by another disease

Measles, Mumps, and Rubella

- ✓ Non-immunization of children
- ✓ Non-immunization of adults
- ✓ Non-immunization of adults whose immunity has waned

Figure 1-2

© 1996 OnGUARD, Inc.

Officers Have a Duty to Protect Themselves and Others

A Denver, Colorado police officer who received a deep bite on his hand while subduing an assault suspect stated:

> "Being bit or spit on doesn't change my basic approach to the job. There's no time to worry first about infection when responding to someone in need of help. I don't have that luxury. If somebody's down there bleeding, I'm going to take the risk that I have to take."[6]

You may share this sentiment. However, while taking time to put on gloves or taking other precautions during an emergency may seem unrealistic, opportunities may present themselves more often than anticipated. The bottom line is that even in an emergency you have to balance your duty to protect the public against your duty to protect yourself. Communicable diseases can have a life changing

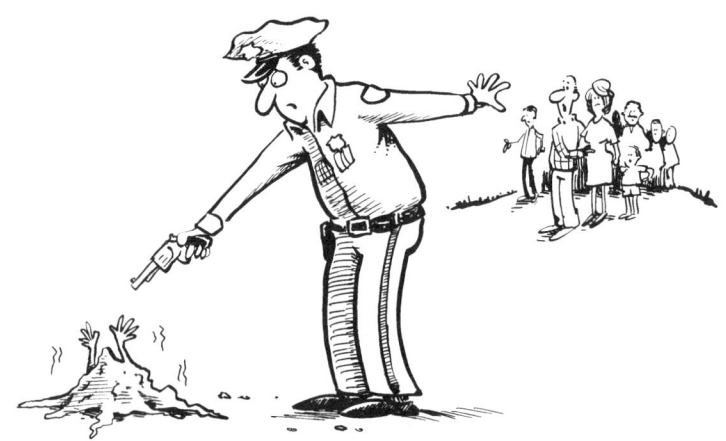

Protect Yourself and Others

© 1996 OnGUARD, Inc.

impact on those who become infected. HIV infection and hepatitis B, in particular, can cause friends and coworkers to shun infected individuals out of fear of contracting the disease themselves. A communicable disease can result in extensive time loss from work due to physical illness and deterioration. Workers' compensation disability benefits may be denied if an exposure cannot be proved to have occurred on the job. The emotional and financial effects of a communicable disease upon family members and loved ones can be far reaching as well.

> **Communicable diseases can have a life changing impact on those who become infected.**

From an ethical standpoint, you also have an obligation to protect coworkers and bystanders at an emergency scene from communicable diseases. Everyone involved with subjects at an emergency scene is at risk of exposure. In light of this fact, it's important to try to limit the number of people having direct contact with subjects.

As with the general public, you may also need to protect emergency victims from communicable diseases. Don't just look at such individuals as a potential source of diseases. Subjects may have weakened immune systems as a result of sickness or open wounds. They may thus be more susceptible to diseases than other people and may be at risk of being infected by you or by someone else at the emergency scene. If you have a cold or some other illness, you might unnecessarily expose subjects to a communicable disease.

Take time to inform yourself about communicable diseases. Otherwise, you may not know what risks are present or how to minimize those risks. You may act out of misinformed fear rather than knowledge in dealing with the possible presence of a communicable disease. Such fear can adversely affect the level and quality of service provided by a law enforcement agency. For example, fear of infection may be revealed in the way you touch or refuse to touch the people you deal with. Attitudes may also be revealed if you use unnecessary and excessive precautions. You need to strike a balance in protecting yourself and others, while still being sensitive to the subjects you deal with, so they won't feel embarrassed or alienated. Education can relieve much of the apprehension you may have in facing communicable diseases.

> **Misinformed fear regarding communicable diseases can adversely affect the level and quality of service provided.**

Once you know how to prevent the spread of communicable diseases, you may be able to provide a valuable educational service in the community. Armed with accurate information, you may have opportunities to instruct various community groups, as well as individuals who are at high risk. You may thus be able to encourage behavior change and reduce the transmission of communicable diseases in your community.

Developing Legal Issues

There are numerous legal issues relating to communicable diseases that you need to be aware of. We'll list them here and then will expand on them in Session 6.

- Withholding police services because of a person's suspected or proven infection status is not permitted.

- Agencies' policies should be consistent with standards and guidelines set forth by the Occupational Safety and Health Administration (OSHA) and the Centers for Disease Control and Prevention (CDC).

- Workers who become infected with a communicable disease on the job and who are still able to perform their job assignments may not be terminated solely because of their disease status.
- Confidentiality of a person's disease status must be balanced against valid needs for disclosure of this information.
- The Ryan White Act sets forth a process by which emergency responders can be notified of a patient's disease status in certain instances.
- Documentation about any exposure incident is critical for obtaining workers' compensation benefits.
- Every law enforcement department should receive training about communicable diseases.
- In many prisons, issues such as mass screening for HIV and segregation of infected inmates must be addressed.

The legal issues relating to communicable diseases are still in the developmental stages. Laws aren't uniform, and there has been considerable diversity in the outcome of civil actions against officers. Barring some extraordinary degree of negligence, your risk of being sued **successfully** is probably not as great as your risk of exposure to a communicable disease. Focus on learning as much as you can about infection control and on putting the information into practice, and you shouldn't need to be overly concerned about being named as a defendant in a civil action.

> **Officers should focus on putting infection control information into practice.**

© 1996 OnGUARD, Inc.

Summary

The importance of training for law enforcement personnel in preventing the spread of communicable diseases cannot be overemphasized. Statistics provide grim evidence of the continuing spread of HIV infection and hepatitis B in the United States. In addition, diseases such as tuberculosis, measles, and other illnesses which were once nearly eradicated have been on the rise in recent years.

Because of the increasing prevalence of communicable diseases in the general population, and because you as a peace officer frequently deal with individuals who are at high risk of being infected, you face a substantial risk of being exposed to these silent assailants on the job. If you try to avoid dealing with individuals suspected or known to have a communicable disease, you may find yourself subject to disciplinary action by your department, and you may become entangled in civil litigation.

You have a duty to protect yourself from communicable diseases, even in extreme emergencies. You also have a duty to protect other people—family members, coworkers, the subjects you deal with, and the community you serve. Training in the ways communicable diseases are spread and in specific steps that you can take to reduce the risk of infection can help you overcome your concerns and act knowledgeably and sensitively in each situation. Federal, state, and local laws regarding infection control, together with various court rulings, must all be taken into account so as to avoid civil liability.

References and Recommended Reading

1. Centers for Disease Control. (1992). *Tuberculosis in correctional facilities* (Narrative text, p. 9; Facsimile of slides, p. 33). Washington, DC: U.S. Government Printing Office.
2. Centers for Disease Control and Prevention. (1995, June). AIDS cases, case-fatality rates — United States, June 1981 – June 1995. *HIV/AIDS Surveillance Report, 7*(1), p. 14.
3. Refresher class: Hepatitis B (1992). *Emergency Medical Services, 21*(8), pp. 64-65.
4. Centers for Disease Control. (1992, April 17). Prevention and control of tuberculosis in U.S. communities with at-risk minority populations: Recommendations of the Advisory Council for the Elimination of Tuberculosis. *Morbidity and Mortality Weekly Report, 41*(RR-5), pp. 1-5.
5. West, K. (1991). The TB comeback. *Emergency Medical Services, 20*(9), pp. 63-66.
6. Ensslin, J. C. (1990, September 30). Cops more likely to face a killer—AIDS. *Rocky Mountain News*, p. 8.

Notes

SESSION 2
Understanding the Silent Assailant

In the last session, we presented statistics demonstrating how communicable diseases have been increasing in prevalence over the last several years. We also pointed out that as a peace officer, you face an increased risk of being exposed to a contagious disease on the job, and we stressed the importance of getting training in preventing the spread of disease.

> **Preventing infection starts with understanding how communicable diseases are spread.**

Before you can take preventive actions, you need to understand how a communicable disease—the silent assailant—causes infection. In this session, we'll start by discussing the elements that must be present before a communicable disease can spread from one person to another. After laying a foundation, we'll give an overview of things you can do to keep from being exposed or becoming infected.

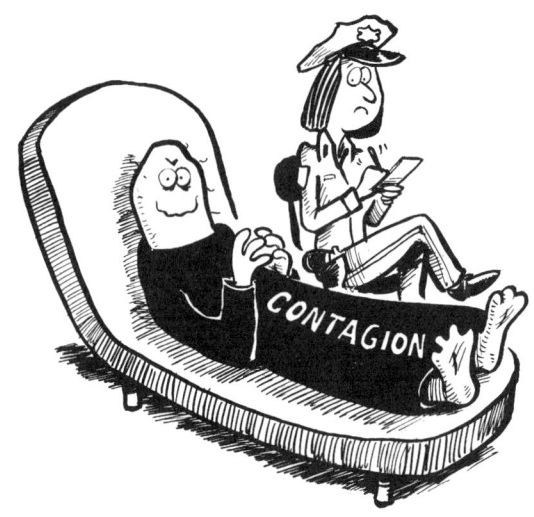

Understand the Silent Assailant

> **OBJECTIVE: State how communicable diseases are spread.**

Key Points

1. A disease can only be transmitted when an *infectious agent* is present.

2. Two ways that an infectious agent can be transmitted from one person to another are through *bloodborne* and *airborne pathogens.*

3. Infectious agents enter the body through a *portal of entry.*

4. There are **factors that make a person more susceptible** to coming down with a disease after being exposed.

5. As a law enforcement officer, you must understand and practice **body substance isolation.**

Certain conditions must be present before a communicable disease can be passed on. Each of the factors listed below is a link in what is called the ***chain of disease transmission:***
- presence of an infectious agent
- efficient mode of transmission
- presence of a portal of entry into the body
- susceptible receiving host

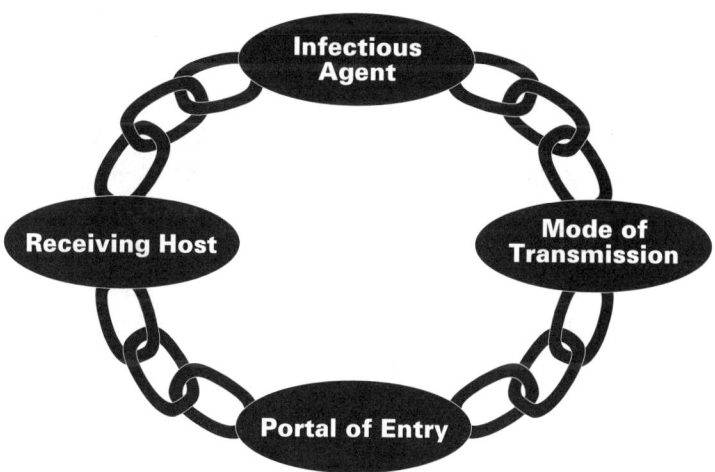

Figure 2-1. Chain of Disease Transmission

Infectious Agent

An **infectious agent** is an organism that causes a disease. In humans, infectious agents are usually either viruses or bacteria. Each infectious agent possesses its own degree of infectability, known as **virulence**, which makes some diseases more infectious than others. The hardiest or most virulent organisms are those that can survive in either the body or the environment. Hepatitis B virus, for example, can survive for at least seven days, dried at room temperatures, on environmental surfaces.[1] It is thus possible for hepatitis B to be spread merely through contact with contaminated surfaces, such as bloodstained equipment or clothing, even if the bloodstain is dried.

> **Hepatitis B can be spread through contact with bloodstained equipment or clothing.**

Organisms with a lower virulence generally cannot survive for more than a few hours in the environment. Tuberculosis (TB) bacteria, for instance, die when exposed to ultraviolet light and air. Low virulence diseases such as TB are not risk free, however. Frequent and prolonged exposure, such as by living or working with infected individuals, increases a person's risk of becoming infected over time.

The **dose**, or number of live infectious organisms present in body fluids, also affects disease transmission. Communicable diseases with high levels of infectious organisms are more readily transmitted even if the exposure involves only a small amount of infected body fluid. For example, depending on the type of exposure, the rate of transmission of hepatitis B virus is normally higher than that of HIV. A person experiencing a single needlestick exposure from someone infected with hepatitis B virus has a 6% to 30% chance of contracting hepatitis B. In contrast, an individual receiving a single needlestick exposure from a person infected with HIV has only a 0.5% chance (1 chance in 200) of contracting HIV. The difference in the rate of transmission is believed to be due to the fact that hepatitis B virus has a higher concentration of infectious organisms in body fluids than HIV.[2]

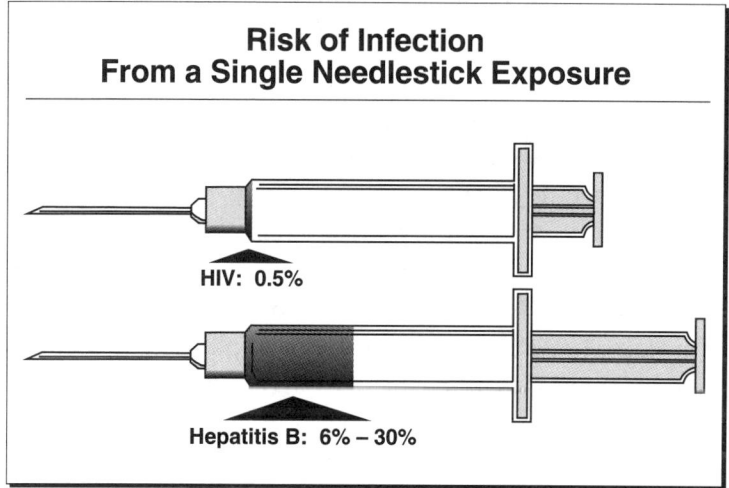

Figure 2-2

Mode of Transmission

The second link in the chain of disease transmission is the *mode of transmission*, or the way an infectious agent moves from one person to another. The mode of transmission may be either bloodborne or airborne, depending on whether the disease organisms are normally spread via the bloodstream or in the air.

Bloodborne Pathogens

Bloodborne pathogens are microorganisms found in human blood that can cause disease in humans. Hepatitis B virus is an example of a bloodborne pathogen. Diseases caused by bloodborne pathogens are known as ***bloodborne diseases***. Besides hepatitis B, other bloodborne diseases include HIV, syphilis, hepatitis C, malaria, and certain types of herpes.

Bloodborne diseases can be spread in several ways. The most risky type of exposure is contact of the blood of an infected person with the blood of another person by means of a puncture wound such as a needlestick. Transmission can also occur when the blood of an infected person contacts a cut, abrasion, chapped area, rash, or other area of damaged skin on another person, or when blood splashes onto the mucous membranes of the eyes, nose, or mouth of another individual. For hepatitis B, blood to blood transmission is most common, but blood to mucous membrane transmission is also possible.

The Centers for Disease Control and Prevention (CDC) has ranked the risk of infection from bloodborne pathogens by mode of transmission. This information is presented in Figure 2-3, with the risk level increasing from bottom to top. As you can see, a needlestick injury carries the greatest risk of infection, with decreasing risk for cuts by contaminated objects, contact with breaks in the skin, and contact with mucous membranes.

© 1996 OnGUARD, Inc.

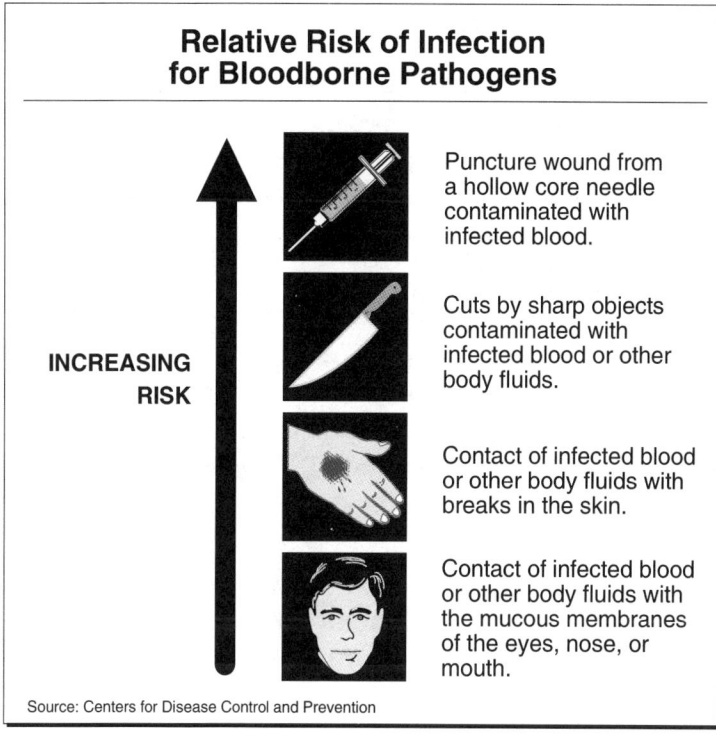

Figure 2-3

Still another way bloodborne diseases can be spread is through cross contamination, in which blood from an infected individual contaminates an object, and then another person is exposed through contact with that object. This route of transmission should be of special concern to you when you are cleaning up body fluids or collecting evidence. Note that bloodborne diseases are **not** transmitted through casual contact. You can't "catch" HIV as you would catch a common cold or the flu.

Airborne Pathogens

Airborne pathogens are disease causing organisms, such as TB bacteria, that are concentrated in saliva and mucus. They are spread when an infected person coughs, sneezes, or exhales infectious droplets onto another person or object. These droplets are so small that they are nearly invisible to the naked eye. They can remain airborne long enough to be inhaled by another person, resulting in disease transmission.

Airborne diseases are often acquired by living or working in the same household or facility with infected individuals, especially if the ventilation system in the building is poor. This problem can be particularly acute in prisons, where many inmates and staff may be exposed to tuberculosis. Besides TB, other airborne diseases include meningitis, mumps, measles, rubella, and chicken pox.

> **Airborne diseases can be spread by living or working in the same facility with infected individuals.**

Portal of Entry

The third link in the chain of disease transmission is the ***portal of entry***, or the way disease organisms get inside the body. There are several possible entryways:

- the bloodstream, via a needlestick through the skin
- breaks in the skin as a result of chapping, abrasions, cuts, lesions, or oozing rash
- the respiratory tract
- the mucous membranes of the eyes, nose, and mouth
- the digestive tract
- the reproductive/urinary tract

© 1996 OnGUARD, Inc.

If an infected body fluid comes in contact with a portal of entry, then the risk of disease transmission is greatly increased.

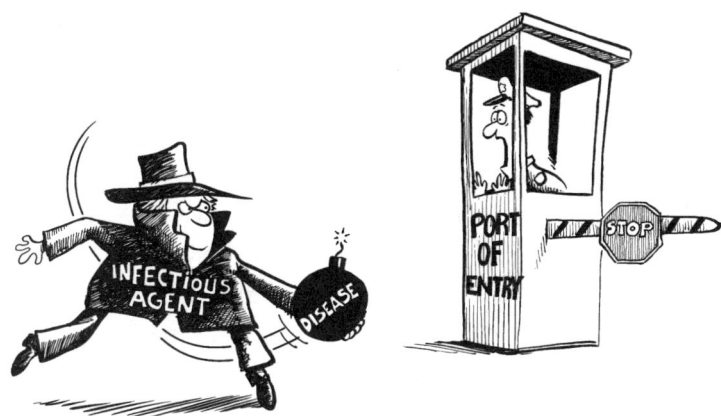

Keep Infectious Agents Away From Any Portal of Entry

Receiving Host

The final link in the chain of disease transmission is the ***receiving host***, or person exposed to the disease. Before disease transmission is complete, infectious organisms must find a host in which they can survive and reproduce. The overall health of the receiving host, including the state of the host's immune system, is a factor in determining the risk of becoming infected after an exposure. When the receiving host is in good health, the body's natural defense mechanisms may be able to ward off infectious organisms. However, when the receiving host's immune system is weakened by another disease or by fatigue, the risk of infection developing from an exposure increases.

It is of utmost importance that you be able to apply the theory from the classroom to the reality of your working environment. One application area relates to the material just presented on the chain of disease transmission. All of the links in the chain of transmission—infectious agent, mode of transmission, portal of entry, and receiving host—must be present before a communicable disease will spread. It therefore follows that if you can remove or diminish one or more of the links, there will be less likelihood of disease transmission. At the scene of an emergency, you should always be looking for ways to break the chain of transmission.

> **Be alert for ways that you can break the chain of disease transmission.**

Body Substance Isolation

Body substance isolation (BSI) is an infection control strategy that can help you break the chain of disease transmission and prevent the spread of communicable diseases. Because of the risk level of disease transmission at any emergency scene, it's mandatory that you practice BSI any time you are dealing with emergency victims. Two cornerstones of BSI should be forever ingrained in your mind:

- **You must treat every individual as if he or she has a communicable disease.**

  There is no way to judge positively from outward appearances whether or not a person has HIV, hepatitis B, tuberculosis, or any other disease. Many infected individuals, especially those with HIV, show no symptoms whatsoever. Subjects may not know their communicable disease status, or if they do know, they may not disclose it to you when asked. They may provide misleading information instead, in order to receive better treatment or other favorable considerations. You can't rely on what subjects tell you. Neither can you rely on subjects' apparent economic level or age as an indicator of the presence of a communicable disease. With so little verifiable information available, the only practical solution is to treat **all** individuals as if they are infected. At the same time, you need to treat everyone with respect, dignity, and compassion. The possible presence of a communicable disease doesn't override basic principles of caregiving and public service.

> **Treat all subjects and all body fluids as if they are infectious.**

- **Treat all body substances as if they are infected with HIV, hepatitis B, or other bloodborne pathogens.**

    It's quite unlikely that you could acquire a bloodborne disease such as HIV or hepatitis B through contact with saliva, respiratory secretions, sweat, tears, vomit, urine, or feces. However, these body fluids may carry other disease organisms, or they could have traces of blood in them, so it's a good idea to take precautions to protect yourself. In addition, several other body fluids may also be infectious. These fluids are listed in Figure 2-4.

© 1996 OnGUARD, Inc.

Potentially Infectious Materials in Addition to Blood

Body Fluids

Amniotic Fluid	The fluid surrounding the fetus in the mother's uterus during pregnancy. It is encountered during childbirth.
Cerebrospinal Fluid	The fluid that circulates in the brain and spinal column. It may leak out when a skull fracture or spinal cord injury has occurred.
Pericardial Fluid	The fluid surrounding the heart. It would normally not be encountered by emergency workers.
Peritoneal Fluid	The fluid surrounding the organs in the abdominal cavity. It may be present when the abdominal wall has been opened and the organs displaced.
Pleural Fluid	The fluid surrounding the lungs. It would normally not be encountered by emergency workers.
Semen	The fluid produced by males upon ejaculation. It may be present at the scene of a sexual assault.
Synovial Fluid	The fluid that lubricates the joints and tendons. It may be encountered when there are compound fractures or joint dislocations.
Vaginal Secretions	Both blood and mucus. Bleeding can occur through menstruation, miscarriage, trauma, or injury to the vaginal wall during sexual activity. Mucous discharge occurs normally, or it may result from an infection. Vaginal secretions may be present after a sexual assault.
Body Fluids Contaminated With Blood	Saliva, vomit, urine, and other fluids. Blood is often evident in these body fluids after a trauma incident.
Unidentifiable Body Fluids	All body fluids should be considered infectious in situations where it is difficult or impossible to differentiate between fluids, as in poorly lighted areas.

Other Substances

Unattached Tissues or Organs	Any unattached tissues or organs from a human, whether the source individual is living or dead. These materials may be encountered at crime scenes, after motor vehicle accidents, and at other major trauma incidents.

Figure 2-4

There is no fail-safe way to identify potentially infectious body fluids and other materials when you're on the job. In most instances, it's impossible to distinguish between infectious and noninfectious body fluids. Emergency situations often involve hostile actions, and they are often poorly lighted. Your ability even to **see** body fluids, much less **identify** them, may be severely limited. For these reasons, when you're working under uncontrolled emergency circumstances, you should treat **all** body fluids as if they are infectious.

BSI involves taking appropriate protective measures whenever there is a risk of exposure to blood or other materials that might be infectious. Specific BSI procedures will be presented and discussed throughout the remainder of this program.

Now that you know how communicable diseases are spread, let's talk about what you can do to protect yourself.

> **OBJECTIVE: Identify general precautions you can take to protect yourself from contracting a communicable disease.**

Key Points

1. Get the **hepatitis B vaccination series** and an annual **TB screening.**

2. Use **personal protective equipment** routinely and dispose of it properly.

3. Take **precautions** immediately **after** any potential **exposure** incident.

4. **Stay healthy** by eating right, exercising regularly, getting enough sleep, etc.

Get Hepatitis B Vaccination and TB Screening

To help prevent the spread of hepatitis B infection, the Occupational Safety and Health Administration (OSHA) has mandated that in the states and jurisdictions falling under its compliance regulations, hepatitis B vaccinations must be made available to all employees having a risk of occupational exposure. The current hepatitis B vaccine is considered one of the safest vaccines ever developed. It is a synthetic product derived from yeast, with no human blood components, so there is no risk of contamination from HIV or other bloodborne pathogens. The vaccine consists of a series of three injections administered over a six month period.

Employers who come under OSHA compliance regulations are required to make hepatitis B vaccinations available free of charge. Future booster doses, if recommended by medical research, must also be free. New employees should be vaccinated within 10 working days of their first assignment where exposure could occur. Although all employees with at-risk assignments are urged to get the hepatitis B vaccination series, they may decline by signing a waiver form. If they change their minds later, OSHA regulations state that they must be allowed to participate in the vaccination program at no cost to themselves. Check with your department if you have any questions about the current hepatitis B vaccination policy for your agency.

> **All officers with at-risk assignments should get the hepatitis B vaccination series.**

There is no vaccine for tuberculosis. However, you can protect yourself from the disease by getting an annual TB screening. The screening should be done using the tuberculin skin test (PPD method). Individuals who show a positive reaction to the test need to be followed up with a chest X-ray or other testing.

It is highly recommended that you get vaccinations for other communicable diseases, such as measles and diphtheria. Figure 2-5 summarizes vaccination recommendations for all law enforcement personnel.

Vaccination Recommendations for All Law Enforcement Officers	
Hepatitis B	Series of three injections with a reevaluation after nine years
Tuberculosis	Yearly screening by PPD method
Diphtheria/Tetanus	Booster every 10 years throughout life
Measles/Mumps/Rubella	Two doses; however, anyone immunized before 1967 should be revaccinated
Polio	One-time dose
Influenza	Yearly dose

Figure 2-5

Use Personal Protective Equipment

Personal protective equipment (PPE) is any equipment or clothing that offers protection for the hands, the body, or the mucous membranes of the eyes, nose, or mouth. Such protective equipment is designed to provide a barrier between you as the wearer and potentially infectious materials. PPE also protects the people you work with from disease organisms that you might be carrying. Gloves, splash resistant eyewear, face masks, protective clothing, and resuscitation equipment are all examples of PPE. OSHA requires employers under its jurisdiction to supply PPE at no cost and in various sizes to employees who are performing tasks in which there is a reasonable expectation of contact with substances that might be infectious.

In evaluating whether to wear PPE, it's helpful to weigh the risks against the benefits in each situation. In the law enforcement profession, the risk of encountering blood or other body fluids is high. Therefore, PPE is strongly recommended for most incidents. Even in emergency situations, the extra seconds it takes to put on PPE are well spent, compared with the consequences of contracting a communicable disease.

> **Personal protective equipment can help reduce the risks you face in emergency situations.**

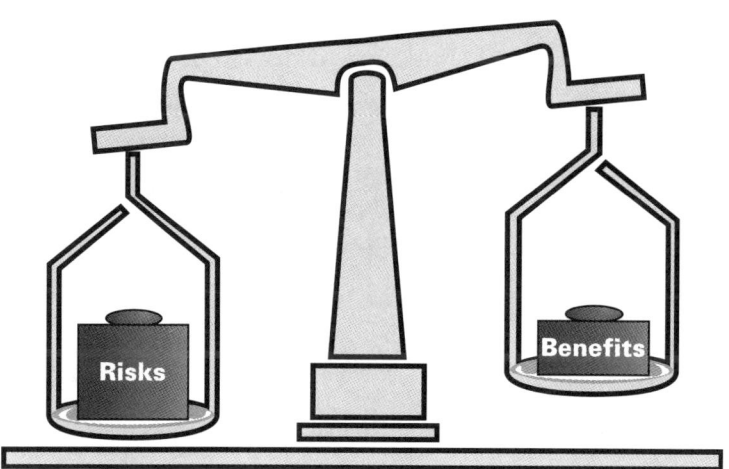

Figure 2-6. Weigh Risks Against Benefits

© 1996 OnGUARD, Inc.

PPE is such an important part of infection control that we'll spend a significant amount of time discussing it in the sessions that follow. For now, just remember that PPE can help cut down on the risks that you face in emergency situations. It can also make subjects feel more at ease, knowing they're protected from any infectious organisms you might have. It makes sense to use such protective equipment routinely in your job.

Take Precautions After Exposure

No matter how careful you may be, situations will arise in which there just isn't time to put on PPE, or in which PPE gets punctured or torn, and an exposure occurs. In such cases, take the following precautions as soon as possible after the incident:

- Remove all contaminated clothing.
- Wash your hands and any other exposed areas thoroughly.
- Report the incident.
- Get appropriate medical testing and follow-up.

As with PPE, precautions following an exposure are extremely important. We'll discuss them in detail in the sessions that follow.

Stay Healthy

Staying healthy is a final way that you can keep from contracting a communicable disease. Remember, when the body is healthy, the immune system may be able to fight off disease organisms. Without an appropriate receiving host, the chain of disease transmission can be broken.

Here are some common sense activities that can help you stay healthy:

- Eat a balanced diet.
- Exercise regularly.
- Get plenty of sleep.
- Don't smoke.
- Wash your hands frequently.
- Keep cuts and other areas of damaged skin covered with a clean bandage.

> **When the body is healthy, the immune system may be able to fight off disease organisms.**

Summary

Communicable diseases can be spread only if a chain of disease transmission is present. This chain includes an infectious agent, whose infectability varies with the virulence of the particular disease and with the dose of the organisms; a mode of transmission, which can be either bloodborne or airborne; a portal of entry, which enables the disease organisms to get inside the body; and a receiving host, in which the disease organisms can survive and multiply. Bloodborne diseases are spread primarily through contact of an infected person's blood with either blood, damaged skin, or mucous membranes of another person. Airborne diseases are spread by breathing infectious droplets in the air.

You should always be alert to ways that you can break the chain of disease transmission. One way is by practicing body substance isolation (BSI), which involves treating every individual as if he or she has a communicable disease and treating all body substances as if they are infectious.

Because of the risk of exposure to hepatitis B and tuberculosis, it is recommended that you get the hepatitis B vaccination series and a yearly screening for TB. To protect yourself from contagious diseases on the job, use personal protective equipment (PPE) whenever you think you might be exposed to blood or other body fluids. If there isn't time to put on PPE, or if an exposure occurs in spite of PPE, take steps immediately after the incident to limit the effects of the exposure. Also, make an effort to follow common sense health precautions so you can stay in good physical condition and keep your immune system strong. These precautions and procedures should help you defend yourself against the silent assailant.

References and Recommended Reading

1. Occupational Safety and Health Administration (1991, December 6). 29 CFR Part 1910.1030, Occupational exposure to bloodborne pathogens: Final rule. *Federal Register, 56*(235), p. 64012.

2. Centers for Disease Control. (1989). *Guidelines for prevention of transmission of human immunodeficiency virus and hepatitis B virus to health-care and public-safety workers* (DHHS Publication No. 89-107), p. 2. Washington, DC: U.S. Government Printing Office.

Notes

SESSION 3
The Balancing Act

Knowledge about communicable diseases and how they're spread is more useful if you can apply the theory to specific situations that you face on the job. To make the application process easier, and to help you balance your duty to protect and serve the public with your duty to protect yourself, we'll present a number of hypothetical situations in the remaining sessions of this program. We'll identify risks to watch out for, appropriate personal protective equipment (PPE) to wear, safe work practices to follow, and personal decontamination procedures to use. In this session, as we get down to specifics, we'll center our discussion around three scenarios: a fight in a cell block, a homicide scene, and a traffic accident scene. The sessions that follow will examine other types of incidents that you might have to deal with in your job.

> It's important for you to be able to apply theory to on the job situations.

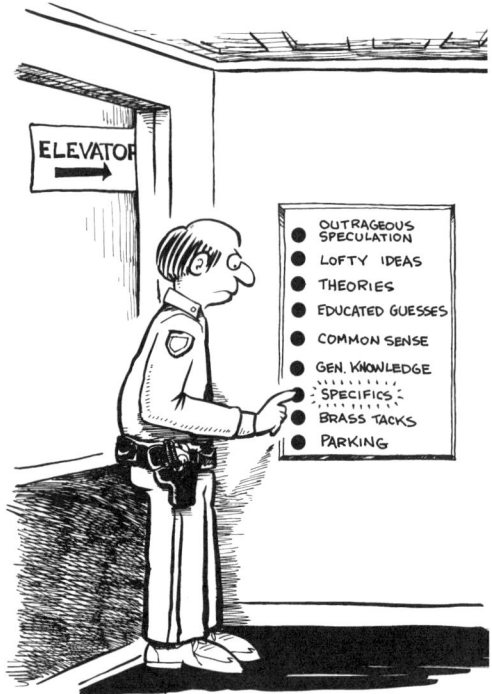

Getting Down to Specifics

Scenario 3-1: Fight in a Cell Block

You're an officer in a detention center. As you pass one of the cell blocks one day, you suddenly hear shouting. You see inmates congregating, but from your present vantage point you can't see exactly what's happening. You call for help and then move in to resolve the situation. As you make your way through the crowd, you notice two inmates fighting. Their faces, hands, and clothing are bloodied. You aren't wearing gloves or other PPE. You intervene and restore order, but in doing so, you get blood on your hands, clothes, and face.

In this scenario, the urgency of the situation probably makes it impractical for you to stop to put on PPE before you intervene in the fight. During the scuffle, you're exposed to blood, which might contain disease organisms. In such a situation, the thing to do is to take steps as soon as possible after the incident to decontaminate yourself and your clothing.

> **OBJECTIVE:** Describe the personal decontamination procedures you should follow if you've been exposed to blood or other body fluids that might be infectious.

Key Points

1. As soon as possible, **remove** any **clothing** that may have come in contact with blood or other body fluids and clean according to departmental regulations and the manufacturer's recommendations.

2. **Wash** your **hands and other skin areas** that may have been exposed.

3. **Cleanse** your **eyes, nose, and mouth,** if exposed.

© 1996 OnGUARD, Inc.

Remove Contaminated Clothing

It's important to remove contaminated clothing as soon as possible after an exposure incident to keep materials that might be infectious from touching your skin. For the incident described in Scenario 3-1, you'll want to change parts of your uniform that were contaminated. Place contaminated clothing in a leakproof plastic bag marked with a biohazard symbol. Finish cleaning yourself up, and then follow your department's and the uniform manufacturer's recommendations for cleaning your uniform. Avoid washing contaminated items at home or at a public laundry. Many agencies contract with a local cleaning company as an alternative. Safe work practices for contaminated laundry are listed in Figure 3-1.

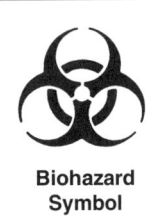

Biohazard Symbol

Safe Work Practices
Contaminated Laundry

- ❖ Handle contaminated laundry as little as possible and by as few people as possible to keep from spreading contaminants.

- ❖ Avoid washing contaminated laundry at home or at a public laundry. A cleaning contract with a private laundry service is a good alternative.

- ❖ If a cleaning service is used, keep contaminated laundry bagged in leakproof bags marked with a biohazard symbol until the items are delivered for cleaning.

- ❖ Follow departmental regulations on disposal of items that are too grossly contaminated to be laundered effectively.

Figure 3-1

Wash Hands and Skin

After you've removed any contaminated clothing, wash your hands and other skin areas that may have come in contact with blood or other body fluids. The Centers for Disease Control and Prevention (CDC) has stated that handwashing is the single most important means of preventing the spread of communicable diseases. The need for proper and frequent handwashing cannot be overemphasized.

> **Handwashing is the single most important means of preventing the spread of communicable diseases.**

If you're responding to an emergency situation away from the station or facility, it's highly recommended that you perform hand and skin washing at the emergency scene as soon as contact with subjects is finished. The longer an area is exposed to substances that might be infectious, the greater the risk of disease transmission. If there isn't any water available at the emergency scene, use disinfectant gel, alcohol towelettes, or a 1 to 100 bleach to water solution for washing. Such cleaners should be stocked in the police vehicle and also within the department. As soon as you can, thoroughly rewash your hands and exposed skin areas using soap and warm running water.

Use either liquid or granular soap for handwashing, if you can. Bar soap tends to hold contaminants and can lead to cross contamination. Perform handwashing even if you were wearing gloves during the incident and even if the gloves appear unpunctured or uncontaminated. It's impossible to see disease organisms with the naked eye, and it's better to take precautions rather than risk disease transmission. In Scenario 3-1, since you weren't wearing gloves, be especially thorough as you wash up.

© 1996 OnGUARD, Inc.

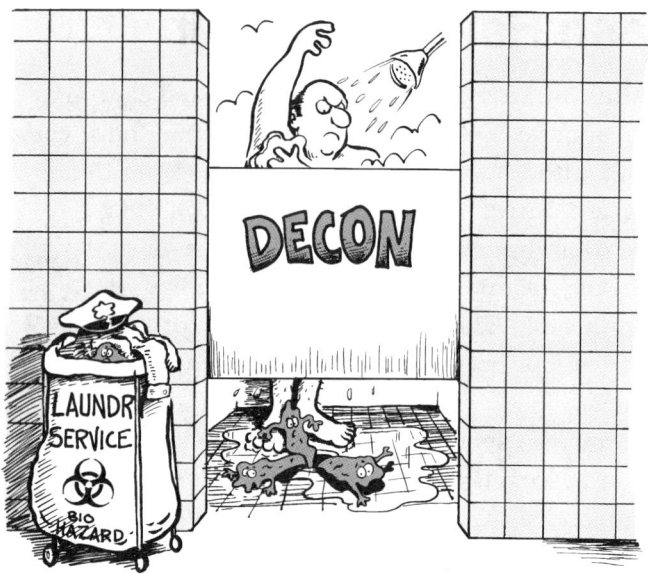

Perform Personal Decontamination

Cleanse Eyes, Nose, and Mouth

If body fluid comes into direct contact with your eyes, nose, or mouth, take steps as soon as possible to remove contaminants. If your eyes are involved, thoroughly rinse them with running water. If your nose is involved, blow into a tissue, and then flush your nostrils with water. If your mouth is involved, spit out any saliva or other fluids, and then rinse your mouth repeatedly with water. All of these procedures may be needed in Scenario 3-1, depending on the extent of contamination.

> **Scenario 3-2: Homicide Scene**
>
> You have responded to an incident in which someone was reported stabbed, and the suspect left the scene in a red pickup truck. When you arrive at the scene, you find a male victim with numerous stab wounds to his neck and abdomen, lying dead on the kitchen floor. There are bloodied footprints throughout the house. Looking around, you notice a bloodied knife lying on the hallway floor. There is a smoldering cigarette in an ashtray on a table, along with some partially eaten food. The house is quiet, and no one else is around.

OBJECTIVE: Identify infection control concerns you should have when entering a crime scene.

Key Points

1. **Protect yourself** from exposure to a communicable disease.
2. Be careful that you **don't spread blood or other body fluids** about the scene.
3. **Guard against exposing others.**

Protect Yourself

In Scenario 3-2, the report indicated that the suspect fled from the scene. Upon arrival, you would want to conduct a search of the premises to verify that no one is present. Then you can proceed with the crime scene investigation. Typically, in such a situation you have time to take precautions to safeguard yourself against exposure to a communicable disease. Don't pass up this opportunity! The risk of exposure is high at incidents such as homicides, assaults, and rapes, because blood and other body fluids are often spread throughout the scene of the crime. Wearing personal protective equipment is your first line of defense. We'll discuss specific items of PPE in a minute. For now, just remember that you need to use PPE whenever possible to protect yourself. It's also essential that you remain consistently diligent as you investigate the crime. An exposure can occur inadvertently if you let your guard down.

> **Wearing personal protective equipment is your first line of defense against communicable diseases.**

Don't Spread Body Fluids

With blood and possibly other body fluids present at the crime scene, it's easy to come in contact with these potentially infectious materials accidentally. You need to be extremely cautious as you move about, paying constant attention to where you step and what you touch. Planning your movements ahead of time can help you avoid splashes, spatters, and unintentional contact with body fluids.

In Scenario 3-2, blood is evident on the victim's body, the floor, and the knife. Saliva and other body fluids may be present on the cigarette. In other situations, depending on the particular crime, clothing, bedding, carpets, walls, and other areas may be contaminated. Body fluids from both the victim and the suspect may be present.

Be aware that dried or partially dried blood and other body fluids may be difficult to see, thus increasing the risk of accidental contact. If contact occurs, there's a good chance that you'll spread body fluids to other parts of the crime scene as you move around. This is particularly true if you aren't aware that you've touched or stepped in anything. Deliberate, careful movements are needed at all times while you're on-scene.

Don't Expose Others

If you've unknowingly come in contact with blood or other body fluids, you may not only contaminate other areas of the crime scene, but you may also expose other people as you interact with them and touch them. As a precaution, you might want to refrain from touching anyone else, if possible, until you've had a chance to remove PPE and contaminated clothing and wash your hands. Also, if there's a chance you might have been exposed to blood or other body fluids at a crime scene, wash your hands and face with soap and water and rinse your eyes with water as soon as practical after leaving the scene, so as to reduce the risk of disease transmission to yourself.

> You may expose others by touching them with contaminated hands or clothing.

© 1996 OnGUARD, Inc.

Now, let's talk about PPE. You know you're supposed to use personal protective equipment, but what do you use, and when?

> **OBJECTIVE:** Given a specific situation, determine whether personal protective equipment should be used and, if so, what type.

Key Points

1. Wear **gloves** whenever **contact with blood or other body fluids** is likely.

2. Use **eye protection, face masks, shoe coverings,** and **body covering** when other parts of your body might come in contact with blood or other body fluids.

3. **Cover** any personal **cuts, abrasions, wounds,** or other areas of **damaged skin** with a clean bandage.

Wear Gloves

In Scenario 3-2, blood is obvious everywhere you look. Since blood and other body fluids may carry disease organisms, the wise course of action is for you to put on gloves immediately upon arrival at the crime scene. As a general rule, any time there's a reasonable chance that you might touch blood or other body fluids, put on disposable gloves before proceeding. It may be useful to keep gloves in a uniform pocket or in a pouch attached to your belt so they'll be readily accessible. Have spare gloves available in your vehicle at all times and on yourself too, if possible.

Disposable gloves aren't tear proof or puncture proof. If you have an open wound on your hands or if you're doing things that involve extensive contact with blood and other body fluids, consider wearing two pairs of gloves for greater protection. If a glove tears during use, change gloves immediately.

Any body fluids you touch while wearing gloves can be transferred from the gloves to other objects. It's important to be careful what you touch while wearing gloves, since contaminants can be spread in this way. Figure 3-2 summarizes safe work practices to follow while wearing gloves.

> **Any body fluids you touch while wearing gloves can be transferred from the gloves to other objects.**

© 1996 OnGUARD, Inc.

Safe Work Practices
Gloves

❖ Carry gloves in a uniform pocket or belt pouch. Have spare gloves in your vehicle and also on your person, if feasible.

❖ Wear correct glove size.

❖ If you wear rings or have long fingernails, use extra care when putting on gloves to avoid tearing gloves.

❖ Change gloves immediately if gloves become torn while being put on or during use.

❖ If possible, change gloves each time you deal with a different person to reduce the risk of cross contamination.

❖ Adjust the type of gloves to fit the situation. For example, use more durable gloves if excessive body fluids are present. Use heavy duty leather gloves if sharp edges are present.

❖ If you wear cotton gloves while collecting evidence, wear latex or vinyl gloves underneath to protect yourself from body fluids.

❖ Don't touch your eyes, nose, or mouth while wearing contaminated gloves. These areas provide disease organisms with a direct route into the body.

❖ Don't handle contact lenses or apply cosmetics or lip balm while wearing gloves.

❖ Be careful what you touch while wearing gloves so you don't spread contaminants.

❖ Remove gloves before eating, drinking, or smoking.

❖ Remove contaminated gloves before entering the cab of the police vehicle.

❖ Remove contaminated gloves before touching personal items such as combs, pens, or eyeglasses to prevent these items from becoming agents of cross contamination.

❖ Dispose of gloves in accordance with departmental regulations. Never leave contaminated gloves at an emergency scene or dispose of them in ordinary trash containers.

❖ Never wash your hands while wearing gloves. Soap breaks down the glove material and lets fluid soak through to your skin.

❖ Never try to rinse and reuse disposable gloves.

❖ Wash your hands thoroughly after removing gloves.

Figure 3-2

© 1996 OnGUARD, Inc.

Use Other PPE

We recommend that you wear PPE such as eye protection, face masks, shoe coverings, and body covering if it's likely that your eyes, nose, mouth, or other parts of your body might be exposed to blood or other body fluids. It's better to put on protective equipment in anticipation of problems than to wish you had after it's too late.

A combination of protective eyewear to shield the eyes and a face mask to cover the nose and mouth gives the best protection for the face. Wear face and eye protection any time spatters or splashes of blood or other body fluids are probable. Dried blood can still be infectious (the hepatitis B virus, for example, can survive for at least one week when dried at room temperature[1]), so it's a good idea to wear face and eye protection if you need to scrape up dried blood samples while collecting evidence.

> **Wear face and eye protection while collecting dried blood samples.**

Figure 3-3 gives safe work practices associated with personal protective equipment for the face and eyes. For the incident described in Scenario 3-2, face and eye protection are recommended, at least while you're collecting evidence, since blood spatters can occur during this process. Shoe coverings are also advisable because of the blood that has been tracked around the crime scene.

Body covering such as gowns, aprons, jackets, and coveralls may be inconvenient, but these items still provide protection when excessive body fluids are present. Appropriate coverings should be kept in the police vehicle and should also be readily available at the station or correctional facility. In Scenario 3-2, due to the amount of blood present, you should wear body covering if you need to remove the victim's body.

© 1996 OnGUARD, Inc.

**Safe Work Practices
Face and Eye Protection**

❖ Wear a face mask and eye protection together for complete shielding of the mucous membranes of the eyes, nose, and mouth.

❖ If you wear prescription eyeglasses, wear additional approved eye protection over them. All protective eyewear should have solid side shields to prevent substances from entering the eyes from the sides.

❖ Wear a face mask and eye protection when dealing with individuals who have an active cough, projectile vomiting, or a suspected respiratory disease.

❖ When dealing with a person who has a productive cough or who is spitting, consider placing a face mask over the individual's mouth and nose. However, don't place a mask on someone if it could interfere with the person's airway.

Figure 3-3

Cover Damaged Skin

Cuts, abrasions, wounds, and other areas of damaged skin can allow disease organisms to get inside the body easily. Because of the risk of disease transmission, it's important to keep such areas covered with a clean dressing while on duty. Check yourself before going on duty each day. Don't overlook small injuries such as nicks, hangnails, and chapped skin. Wear gloves or other PPE over any dressings to reduce further the chance of disease transmission.

In addition to the risks posed by the blood at the crime scene in Scenario 3-2, the knife is also a source of danger. Sharp objects such as knives, syringes with needles, drug paraphernalia, and broken glass are collectively referred to as **sharps**. As a law enforcement officer, you encounter these items frequently. It's important that you know how to handle them safely for infection control purposes.

> ***OBJECTIVE: Identify proper procedures for handling needles and sharp evidence.***

Key Points

1. ***Handle needles safely.***

2. Use a ***puncture resistant container*** for disposing of sharps and for collecting sharp evidence.

Handle Needles Safely

The most common occupational exposure for emergency response personnel is through a needlestick. Research has shown that 80% of HIV and hepatitis B infections acquired on the job are caused by needlestick exposures.[2] To reduce the chance of getting a needlestick, make it a habit not to handle needles at all except to place them in a container for disposal or evidence collection. Don't leave needles stuck into objects or lying around the emergency scene, and don't try to recap, break, or otherwise manipulate needles. Just put them in an appropriate container.

Use a Puncture Resistant Container

Place any needles and other sharp objects that you find at the scene of an emergency directly in a puncture resistant container, or **sharps container**, in order to reduce the chance of accidental injuries. The container should be leakproof on the sides and bottom. There should be a tight fitting lid to prevent spillage and to keep the contents from protruding through the opening. It's a good idea to carry at least two sharps containers in the police vehicle at all times. Use one for sharps that you want to dispose of. Use the other for sharp items that may be needed as evidence. Be sure to label any evidence containers appropriately.

> The use of sharps containers can help reduce accidental injuries.

In Scenario 3-2, you'll want to save the knife as evidence. Wearing gloves, pick up the knife according to accepted crime scene procedures and place it in a clean, unused sharps container to take back to the lab. If the knife is too large to fit in a sharps container, securely protect the blade and the entire instrument in accordance with accepted crime scene procedures before removing the knife from the scene. Figure 3-4 summarizes safe work practices for handling and disposing of sharps.

© 1996 OnGUARD, Inc.

Safe Work Practices Handling Sharps

- Needles should **never** be:
  - ✓ recapped
  - ✓ purposely bent or broken by hand
  - ✓ removed from disposable syringes
  - ✓ manipulated by hand

- Never dispose of sharps in any trash container other than a sharps container.

- Place all sharps directly in a sharps container as soon as possible.

- Always place needles in a sharps container by inserting the needle end first.

- Never force needles or other sharps into a sharps container.

- Never insert your fingers into a sharps container for any reason.

- Dispose of sharps containers in accordance with department policy when the containers are three-fourths full.

- Place items such as knives and drug paraphernalia that may be needed as evidence in a clean, unused sharps container and label appropriately.

- If a sharp edged instrument such as a knife, machete, or axe is needed as evidence and is too large to fit in a sharps container, securely protect the sharp edge and the entire device according to accepted evidence collection procedures before transporting the item. Think about the safety of personnel who will handle the instrument after you do.

- When collecting glass:
  - ✓ Don't pick up pieces with your bare hands. Instead, use some type of tweezers or other device.
  - ✓ Remember that disposable gloves can be easily torn.

Figure 3-4

© 1996 OnGUARD, Inc.

The final risk that is present in Scenario 3-2 is handling a dead body. Precautions are called for here, just as in the rest of the crime scene investigation.

> **OBJECTIVE: Describe the precautions you should follow when handling a dead body.**

Key Points

1. **Don't touch** anything at a crime scene **unless** you're **authorized** to handle evidence.

2. **Follow standard infection control procedures** if you need to touch or remove a corpse, **regardless of** whether the subject is known or suspected to be infected with **HIV.**

Don't Touch

Touching objects can destroy evidence. It can also spread disease organisms if you come in contact with infected body fluids. In Scenario 3-2, there's a substantial amount of blood on and around the victim. Other body fluids may also be present. If the person had a communicable disease, you could easily be exposed while handling the body, and you could spread the infected body fluids and possibly expose others as you move about. To be safe, don't touch anything unless you're authorized to do so.

Use BSI Procedures

If you have authorization to touch or remove a dead body, follow standard **body substance isolation (BSI) procedures** as you work. In other words:

- Cover all personal cuts and abrasions.
- Wear gloves and face/eye protection.
- Wear body covering if you think your body might contact blood or other body fluids.
- Wash all exposed areas after any contact with blood or other body fluids.

It's a good idea to wear full body covering when handling a dead body, even if you don't see much blood on or around the victim. In 1991, a medical examiner in the Dallas, Texas area was called in by the Dallas Police Department to remove a shooting victim from a van. The victim was seat belted into the front passenger seat. He had received multiple gunshot wounds in the back of his head and shoulders, but very little blood was evident. It was estimated that he had been dead for six to nine hours by the time the medical examiner arrived. There was limited space around the van, making it impossible to open the doors fully. The medical examiner was wearing gloves but had no other PPE on. As he pulled the body from the van, he was unable to provide adequate support because of the space limitations, and the body dropped to the ground. Upon impact, a large quantity of blood, which had drained from the body and pooled in the seat of the victim's trousers, burst from the clothing, splattering everywhere. The medical examiner's legs and feet were drenched. He couldn't get out of his clothes fast enough! A neighbor's

> **Full body covering is recommended for handling a dead body.**

garden hose had to be used to help him clean up. His shoes were too contaminated to be cleaned and had to be thrown away.

Incidents like this one point out the need for taking adequate precautions **before** a problem arises. Be sure to use these precautions with **all** victims and **all** body fluids, not just with those you think might be infected with HIV. Remember, HIV isn't the only communicable disease you need to think about. Hepatitis B can also be a killer, and it's much more infectious than HIV. It's impossible to tell just by looking at a person, either living or dead, whether the individual is infected with a communicable disease. You need to follow BSI procedures in **all** circumstances.

Scenario 3-3: Traffic Accident Scene

You've just arrived at the scene of a two car collision. A vehicle heading north on a through street was struck broadside by another car that ran a red light. One of the passengers in the vehicle that was hit is lying on the shoulder of the road, with blood spurting from his arm. The other passenger has face injuries and appears to be going into shock. No one else was injured. The accident occurred on a Tuesday at 5:00 p.m., on a heavily traveled four lane divided highway. Your beat partner helps with traffic while you attend to the injured parties.

As a police officer, you generally don't need to provide extensive emergency medical care, but you may be called on to perform basic first aid or CPR while waiting for medical personnel to arrive. Knowing what personal protective equipment is needed in these situations is an important part of being prepared for such emergencies.

> **OBJECTIVE: List the types of personal protective equipment you should use when giving first aid to a person.**

Key Points

1. *Put on gloves as you approach* the emergency scene. Have *eye protection, a face mask, shoe coverings,* and *body covering* readily available.

2. If resuscitation is needed, use a pocket mask or other *airway device with a one way valve* to keep body fluids from entering your mouth.

Put on Gloves

In Scenario 3-3, the vehicles aren't in danger of catching fire or being hit by other cars. Your life isn't threatened, as it might be in a shooting incident or an assault. Even though both victims are bleeding and need prompt attention, there's still time for you to take precautions to protect yourself before you begin administering first aid.

Your first action should be to put on gloves. Do this quickly as you step out of the police vehicle and approach the emergency scene. In Scenario 3-3, it would be a good idea to carry an extra pair of gloves with you so you can change gloves when you move from one victim to the other.

Even if blood isn't visible, it's recommended that you wear gloves whenever you administer first aid. Other body fluids, such as saliva, vomit, and urine, can contain disease organisms. They can also contain tiny amounts of blood, especially during trauma incidents. To reduce the risk of exposure, you should routinely put on gloves at **every** first aid incident.

> **Wear a face mask, protective eyewear, and body covering if spurting blood is present.**

The presence of spurting blood on one of the victims in Scenario 3-3 should prompt you to put on face and eye protection in addition to gloves, in order to protect your eyes, nose, and mouth. Body covering is also recommended in Scenario 3-3 due to the spurting blood. Even putting on a jacket would be appropriate, provided the jacket is properly cleaned if it gets contaminated.

All items of personal protective equipment should be within easy reach in your vehicle. Another situation that would call for full face and body protection is emergency childbirth, which typically involves large quantities of body fluids.

Use an Airway Device

If you need to perform rescue breathing or CPR, use an airway device such as a disposable pocket mouth to mouth mask. These devices should have a one way valve to prevent the patient's body fluids from entering your mouth. Due to the risk of encountering blood in body fluids, along with the number of diseases that can be transmitted through direct contact with secretions from a person's mouth, you are urged to use traditional mouth to mouth resuscitation only as a last resort.

> **Use traditional mouth to mouth resuscitation only as a last resort.**

Summary

Although the ideal situation is for you to take steps to protect yourself from communicable diseases before you get involved in an emergency situation, in reality it isn't always possible to put on personal protective equipment or take other precautions ahead of time. You need to perform a balancing act—doing your job and yet protecting yourself.

If you're exposed to blood or other body fluids during an emergency incident, decontaminate yourself as soon as possible after the incident to reduce the risk of disease transmission. Decontamination involves removing contaminated clothing, washing your hands and other exposed skin areas, and cleansing your eyes, nose, and mouth, if they were exposed. Handwashing is especially important and should be performed both at the emergency scene and again at the station or facility.

If an emergency situation isn't violent or life threatening to you, take time to use personal protective equipment

© 1996 OnGUARD, Inc.

when dealing with subjects and victims. Put on gloves whenever there's a chance that you might touch blood or other body fluids. Wear protective eyewear and a face mask if spurting blood, spatters of dried blood, or splashes of body fluids are likely to occur. Use shoe coverings and body covering if large amounts of blood or other body fluids are present. Keep any personal cuts or abrasions covered. Use an airway device with a one way valve for resuscitation.

When working at an emergency scene, be watchful of where you step and what you touch, so you don't spread body fluids accidentally. As much as possible, avoid touching other people at the scene to reduce the risk of disease transmission. Unless authorized to handle evidence, try to keep from touching anything that might serve as evidence. Use safe work practices when handling sharp objects, and have puncture resistant containers available for storing or disposing of such items. When handling a dead body, follow body substance isolation procedures, just as with live subjects and with isolated body fluids.

References and Recommended Reading

1. Occupational Safety and Health Administration. (1991, December 6). 29 CFR Part 1910.1030, Occupational exposure to bloodborne pathogens: Final rule. *Federal Register, 56*(235), p. 64012.
2. Marcus, R., & the CDC Cooperative Needlestick Surveillance Group. (1988). Surveillance of health care workers exposed to blood from patients infected with the human immunodeficiency virus. *New England Journal of Medicine, 319*(17), pp. 1118-1123.

SESSION 4

Arrests, Searches, Vehicle Decon

We stressed in the last session that if you can, you should put on gloves and use other **personal protective equipment (PPE)** any time you think you might find blood or other body fluids at an emergency scene. If you don't have time to put on PPE and you happen to come in contact with body fluids, you should remove any contaminated clothing as soon as possible, thoroughly wash your hands and other exposed skin areas, and cleanse your eyes, nose, and mouth, if they were exposed. These protective measures are all part of the strategy of **body substance isolation**, or **BSI**, which emphasizes that all body substances should be treated as if they might be infectious.

BSI applies to situations such as arrests, patdowns, and searches, which you as a peace officer often encounter, but which other emergency response personnel usually don't have to deal with. When you're arresting someone, for

> Practice infection control techniques at all emergency incidents.

example, the suspect might try to spit on you or bite you, or you might find a hypodermic needle hidden in a sock or pocket as you conduct a patdown. You might also encounter hidden needles or knives during a vehicle search. In this session, we'll address these special concerns. We'll also discuss proper procedures for vehicle decontamination.

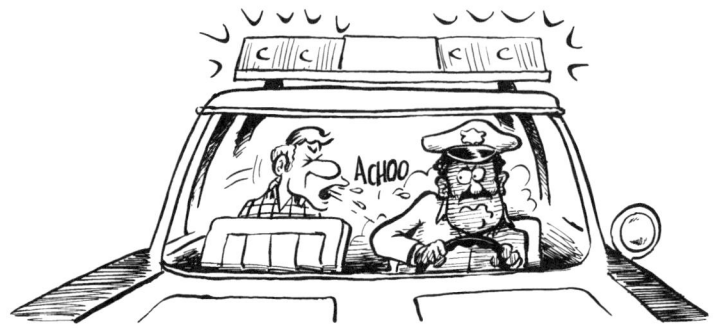

Exposures Can Occur During Arrests

> ### Scenario 4-1: Making an Arrest
>
> *It's 1:00 a.m. Saturday. As you patrol your beat, you observe a car weaving in traffic in an erratic manner. You suspect the driver is intoxicated. You stop the vehicle, and after a roadside sobriety test, you determine you have sufficient cause to arrest the driver for drunk driving. After being handcuffed, the suspect gets angry and starts swearing and spitting at you.*

> **OBJECTIVE: Describe the risk of contracting a communicable disease when arresting a suspect, and state the precautions you should take to minimize the possibility of disease transmission.**

Key Points

1. **Spitting** carries a **low risk** of infection by a communicable disease. To combat spitting, wear **eye protection** and a **face mask,** or place a **mask on the subject. Cleanse** contaminated areas thoroughly.

2. **Biting** is generally **low risk** also. **Cleansing** the wound is an effective follow-up step.

3. **Cuts and needlesticks** are **higher risk** and are possible during **patdowns. Wear gloves, take your time,** and **be careful.**

Spitting

Spitting and biting on the part of arrestees are common concerns for law enforcement personnel. While these behaviors can result in an exposure to a communicable disease, the risk of disease transmission is actually quite low. HIV and the hepatitis B virus occur only in very low concentrations in saliva.[1] As long as there isn't any visible blood in the saliva, and as long as you take appropriate follow-up measures, you don't need to be unduly concerned about contracting a communicable disease.

If someone spits at you, there are three things you can do:

- Put on protective eyewear and a face mask to protect your eyes, nose, and mouth in case the person spits again.

> **Spitting can often be controlled by placing a face mask on the subject.**

- Consider placing a mask over the subject's nose and mouth. Don't do this, though, if the person is drunk and could vomit or if the mask will make breathing difficult.

- Thoroughly wash your hands and any other exposed skin areas as soon as possible after the incident. If your eyes, nose, or mouth were exposed, flush them thoroughly with water.

In Scenario 4-1, since the subject is drunk and could vomit, it's best not to try to put a mask over his nose and mouth. Instead, put protective eyewear and a mask on yourself. After the incident, thoroughly wash any skin areas that were contaminated and properly dispose of or decontaminate any PPE that you used.

Biting

A bite generally won't expose you to infectious organisms. The only way you could get a bloodborne disease through a human bite would be if the subject had infected blood or lesions in his or her mouth before biting you and the infected blood came into contact with your blood, or if disease organisms were present in the subject's saliva and some of the organisms were transferred to your blood through the bite. Both possibilities are remote.

If you get bitten by a person, wash the area thoroughly with soap and warm water, report the incident, and then get medical attention, if necessary.

Patdowns

When conducting a patdown, exercise caution: suspects may place syringes, razor blades, and other sharp objects on their bodies or in their pockets in such a way as to inflict injury upon unsuspecting officers. You might become the victim of a cut, needlestick, or puncture wound if you aren't careful. Follow these suggestions:

- Once you have the suspect under control, take time to put on disposable gloves before proceeding.

- Take your time. The emergency situation should be under your control at this point. Don't rush. Instead, be careful and thorough.

- Before you begin the patdown, ask the suspect if he or she has any concealed needles, knives, or weapons.

- Look before you touch. If you need to pull clothing out of the way, use a flashlight, baton, or other instrument to help you. Don't reach into areas where you can't see what you're doing.

- Keep in mind that disposable gloves aren't puncture proof, but they do provide some protection from cuts and needlesticks. Thicker gloves offer more protection, but they're also more bulky and less effective in locating objects. Agencies should select the thickness of glove that provides the best balance of protection and search efficiency.

> **Disposable gloves aren't puncture proof, but they do provide some protection during patdowns.**

- If blood or other body fluids are evident on the suspect or if you have any cuts or areas of damaged skin on your hands, you might want to consider wearing two pairs of gloves so that you'll have extra protection. Just make sure you can still feel what you're doing if you try double gloving. It may be useful to try wearing two pairs of gloves during other activities or when not on duty to get used to the sensations.

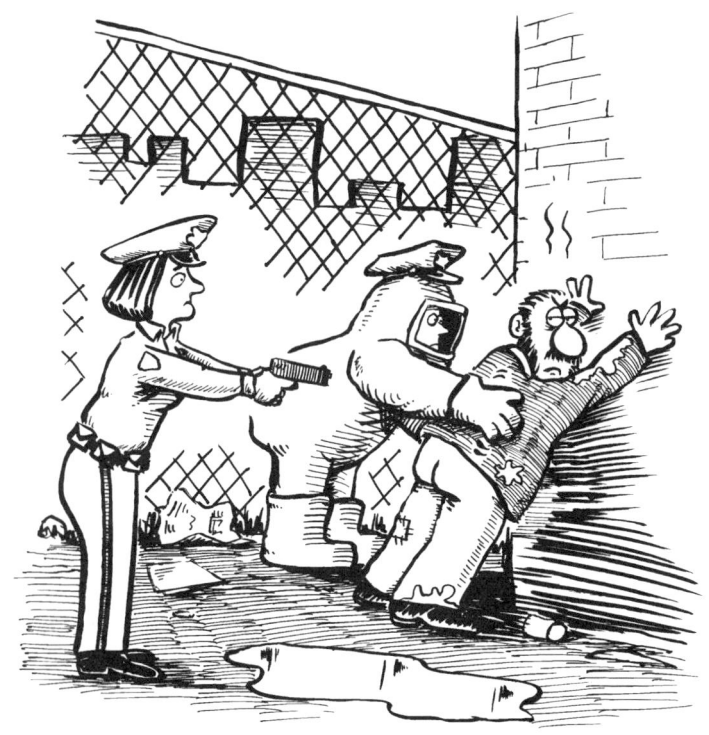

Exercise Caution During Patdowns

Scenario 4-2: Searching a Vehicle

After securing the drunk driver that you arrested in Scenario 4-1, you begin to secure his vehicle. You notice a .45 semiautomatic on the front passenger seat. In checking the weapon, you suspect that it was stolen and that it was used in a robbery. You have the car impounded and transported to the department impound lot for further investigation. At the impound lot, you search the car for evidence related to a robbery.

OBJECTIVE: Identify precautions you should take when conducting a vehicle search to minimize the risk of exposure to a communicable disease.

Key Points

1. Use *personal protective equipment.*
2. *Don't reach without looking.* Use a *flashlight* and a *long handled mirror* to help you.

Use PPE

Vehicle searches are usually done in a controlled environment, in which you have time to put on PPE without endangering yourself. Gloves are a must, since you never know what you might touch. You should also put on body protection if you think you might get body fluids on yourself. If you're working under poor lighting conditions, it's advisable to use body covering whether you can see spills of body fluids or not, so as to have maximum protection.

> **Avoid touching blood and other body fluids even with PPE on.**

Try to avoid touching body fluids even with PPE on. Once you touch blood or other body fluids, you create a risk that you'll spread these substances around when you touch other objects. Don't complicate matters. You have enough to watch out for without adding to the risk of exposure. Stay clear of blood and other body fluids, if possible.

In Scenario 4-2, you'll need gloves for the vehicle search, but you probably won't need body covering, since this was a nonviolent arrest and assuming the impound lot is well lighted.

Look Before Reaching

Most exposures during vehicle searches result from reaching under a seat, into corners, or under the car body without first looking to see what's there. Needles, knives, and other sharp objects are often left on the floor or may be stashed in crevices and corners, so it's important that you work deliberately and take your time while conducting a search. The Centers for Disease Control and Prevention (CDC) recommends using a flashlight, even during daylight

© 1996 OnGUARD, Inc.

hours, along with a long handled mirror to enhance the range of your vision.[2] If you need to move piles of clothing or other objects, use a baton, pen, or other instrument to help you.

Searching a holding cell calls for the same precautions that a vehicle search does. Arrestees may hide contraband in the holding cell before being transferred to the main jail. Be on the lookout for needles, razor blades, and other sharp items, and take time to protect yourself before starting a search.

Scenario 4-3: Vehicle Decontamination

The drunk driver you arrested in Scenario 4-1 vomited in your cruiser on the way to the police station, making it necessary for you to decontaminate your vehicle.

Frequently when you're transporting someone, you'll end up with blood or other body fluids in your vehicle due to injuries sustained or vomiting. Precautions are needed while you're cleaning your vehicle, just as when you're dealing with subjects. Exposures can still occur through contact with body fluids. In this situation, however, if vomit is the only fluid you're dealing with and there's no visible blood in it, the risk of disease transmission is low.

> **OBJECTIVE: Outline proper procedures for decontaminating a vehicle.**

Key Points

1. Use **personal protective equipment** during decontamination.

2. **Soak up** body fluid **spills.**

3. **Preclean** contaminated surfaces with **soap and water.**

4. **Disinfect** surfaces with a 1:100 solution of household **bleach and water** or other EPA registered disinfectant.

5. Allow surfaces to **air dry.**

Use PPE

The latex or vinyl gloves that you wear when dealing with subjects or victims aren't suitable for clean-up operations. For adequate protection during decontamination tasks, you need utility cleaning gloves. If splashes are likely, face and eye protection and body covering are also recommended. In Scenario 4-3, utility gloves, face and eye protection, and body protection are all necessary to minimize the risk.

Soak Up Spills

Soak up spills of blood and other body fluids with paper towels, rags, or other absorbent materials. Dispose of all materials used in the cleaning process in leakproof bags marked with a biohazard symbol, according to departmental regulations. In Scenario 4-3, soak up the vomit and then clean the contaminated surfaces of the vehicle as outlined below.

Preclean

Saturate any dried body fluids with hot soapy water so the surfaces can be cleaned without a lot of scrubbing. Then remove visible contaminants from the interior surfaces of the vehicle by scrubbing thoroughly with soap and hot water. If your hands or clothing were contaminated while you were transporting the subject, be sure to clean the driver's area of the vehicle, including the steering wheel, front seat, and door handles. Use a brush to scrub porous surfaces, such as seatbelts and upholstery. Also use a brush for areas with crevices, such as moldings, to make sure you remove all contaminants. Dispose of soapy water in a floor drain or mop sink.

> **Precleaning surfaces with soap and hot water removes visible contaminants.**

Disinfect

After precleaning with soap and water, wipe or spray surfaces with a bleach solution or other EPA registered disinfectant to disinfect them. Items such as eyeglasses, handcuffs, and other equipment handled during the investigation will also need to be disinfected. Pens and pencils should be disposed of or disinfected as well.

> **Surfaces can be disinfected by wiping or spraying with a bleach solution.**

The Centers for Disease Control and Prevention has indicated that concentrations ranging from one part bleach in 100 parts of water (1:100) up to one part bleach in 10 parts of water (1:10) are effective, depending on the amount of blood, mucus, and other body substances present on the surfaces to be cleaned and disinfected. A 1:10 solution may damage some surfaces with repeated exposure. In most instances, a 1:100 bleach solution should be sufficient. This concentration is equivalent to about 1/4 cup of household bleach in a gallon of tap water. Bleach solutions should be made up fresh daily for best results.[3]

Air Dry

Disinfected areas should be allowed to air dry, if possible. Air drying is important for the following reasons:

- Some organisms die when exposed to air.
- Attempting to dry the surface by wiping it with a drying towel may remove the disinfectant.
- Wiping the surface dry may spread contaminants hidden in crevices or located on the drying towel.

- Surfaces dry more thoroughly in the air than when wiped dry.

Once decontamination is complete, rinse the sponges, brushes, buckets, and other items used for decontamination in a fresh bleach solution. Dispose of any disposable personal protective equipment that you wore during decontamination, according to departmental regulations. Put reusable PPE such as protective eyewear and utility gloves in a designated location to be decontaminated. Be sure to wash your hands before performing any other tasks.

> **Perform handwashing after any cleaning tasks.**

Summary

As a law enforcement officer, you encounter situations not common to other emergency response personnel, such as being spit upon or bitten while arresting suspects or running the risk of needlesticks or cuts during patdowns and vehicle searches. The chance of disease transmission through spitting and biting is low, but it's wise to take precautions anyway. When dealing with spitting, either wear a face mask and eye protection yourself, or place a mask on the subject. Cleanse all exposed areas thoroughly as soon as possible. In the case of a bite, wash the area thoroughly, report the incident, and then follow up with a visit to a medical practitioner. To avoid injury during a patdown, wear gloves and proceed cautiously. When searching a vehicle, wear gloves and, in many cases, body protection. Use a flashlight and long handled mirror to search under seats and in crevices.

© 1996 OnGUARD, Inc.

Wear utility gloves during vehicle decontamination. Face and eye protection and body covering may also be needed. Soak up spills of body fluids first. Then scrub all areas having visible contaminants with hot soapy water. Apply a 1:100 bleach solution to disinfect surfaces, and allow the surfaces to air dry.

References and Recommended Reading

1. Centers for Disease Control. (1989, February). *Guidelines for prevention of transmission of human immunodeficiency virus and hepatitis B virus to health-care and public-safety workers* (DHHS Publication No. 89-107), pp. 10, 32. Washington, DC: U.S. Government Printing Office.

2. Centers for Disease Control. (1989, February). *Guidelines for prevention of transmission of human immunodeficiency virus and hepatitis B virus to health-care and public-safety workers* (DHHS Publication No. 89-107), p. 17. Washington, DC: U.S. Government Printing Office.

3. Centers for Disease Control. (1989, February). *Guidelines for prevention of transmission of human immunodeficiency virus and hepatitis B virus to health-care and public-safety workers* (DHHS Publication No. 89-107), pp. 12, 29, 40. Washington, DC: U.S. Government Printing Office.

SESSION 5
Collecting Evidence

Although much of your work in police services typically involves direct contact with subjects, there are times when you'll be dealing with a "cold" crime scene. The homicide incident discussed in Session 3 (page 45) is an example of this type of situation. As we emphasized in the homicide scenario, you need to take precautions to protect yourself and others from communicable diseases at a crime scene, even though no living subject is present to spread disease organisms. Appropriate actions include wearing personal protective equipment, being careful not to spread blood and other body fluids about the scene, handling needles and other sharp objects safely, and following infection control procedures when handling a dead body.

> **There is a risk of disease transmission even at "cold" crime scenes.**

In this session, we'll look at another type of "cold" crime scene—that of a sexual assault. Three areas will be covered: (1) general precautions to take while on-scene, (2) procedures to follow while collecting evidence, and (3) personal decontamination steps to take when you're finished with your duties. The material in this session is particularly aimed at lab technicians, evidence technicians, and others who collect evidence, but you should find the information useful no matter what your job description may be.

Scenario 5-1: Sexual Assault Scene

You've just arrived at the scene of a sexual assault. You know the victim was beaten and raped repeatedly in several rooms throughout the house. She has already been transported to the hospital for examination, and a suspect has been arrested. Your job is to collect evidence at the scene of the crime.

OBJECTIVE: Outline precautions you should take while investigating a "cold" crime scene.

Key Points

1. **Wear disposable gloves.**

2. **Don't smoke, eat, or drink** while on-scene. **Keep** pencils, fingers, and other **objects out of your mouth** and **away from your face.**

Wear Gloves

As we stressed in the homicide incident, a "cold" crime scene gives you plenty of time to put on personal protective equipment before you start investigating the incident or collecting evidence. Put on gloves as soon as you arrive. Blood and other body fluids may be spattered around the scene and may be difficult to see. In Scenario 5-1, since you know the victim was raped in more than one room of the house, you can anticipate finding semen, blood, and possibly other body fluids in several locations. Gloves will protect you from contacting these potentially infectious materials accidentally. Don't become careless just because the scene is cold. There's still a risk of infection by some communicable diseases, such as hepatitis B, even after body fluids have dried.

Don't Put Things in Your Mouth

Smoking, eating, and drinking at the scene of a crime may seem like harmless activities, but they can result in exposure to a communicable disease. If your hands or gloves are contaminated, disease organisms can easily be transferred to your cigarette, sandwich, soft drink can, or other object when you touch these items. The route of disease transmission is completed when you touch the cigarette, food, or beverage container to your lips.

> **Don't smoke, eat, or drink at the scene of a crime.**

The same risk exists with other objects that you might put in your mouth, such as pencils and pens. The bottom line is that you need to keep **all** objects out of your mouth

© 1996 OnGUARD, Inc.

while you're on-scene. Keep your fingers away from your mouth too, and also be careful not to touch or rub your eyes or nose. Hand to face movements are often performed almost unconsciously. Pay attention to your gestures, and make an effort to break bad habits. You may want to wear a face mask and protective eyewear for added protection. Remember that disease organisms can enter your body through the mucous membranes of your eyes, nose, and mouth. Try not to give such organisms a chance.

We turn now to safe work practices to use during evidence collection.

> **OBJECTIVE: List procedures you should follow when collecting evidence.**

Key Points

1. Wear *personal protective equipment.*

2. Take precautions to *minimize splashing* during collection of wet body fluids. Use *spillproof and leakproof containers* for packaging.

3. Use *tape, not staples,* to seal evidence bags.

4. Use *tweezers* or prongs for picking up *broken glass* or other contaminated sharp items.

5. *Label* all evidence containers clearly, warning of potentially *infectious materials.*

6. Pack evidence **collection tools** in plastic bags and **dispose of or decontaminate** them properly.

Wear Other PPE

You already have gloves on, but often you need additional protection when you start collecting evidence. Choose appropriate PPE according to the tasks you'll be performing. If you need to gather up bedding, put on face and eye protection and body covering before you start, in order to protect yourself from body fluids, both wet and dry. Likewise, use gloves, eye protection, a face mask, and body covering for scraping up blood samples. Remember, dried blood can still be infectious. Particles of dried blood can easily become airborne when a bloodstain is scraped, so you need to make sure your hands, face, and body are protected.

> Use appropriate PPE for gathering up bedding or scraping up dried blood samples.

If you wear cotton gloves when working with items that might have fingerprint value, wear your regular latex or vinyl gloves underneath to protect yourself from body fluids. If there's a chance that you might step in body fluids as you move around, put on shoe coverings so you won't track blood or other body fluids into your vehicle or back to the police station.

In Scenario 5-1, full protection is recommended—gloves, eye protection, face mask, body covering, and shoe coverings—since the assault was carried out in several rooms and since you'll probably need to gather up bedding and scrape up dried blood samples.

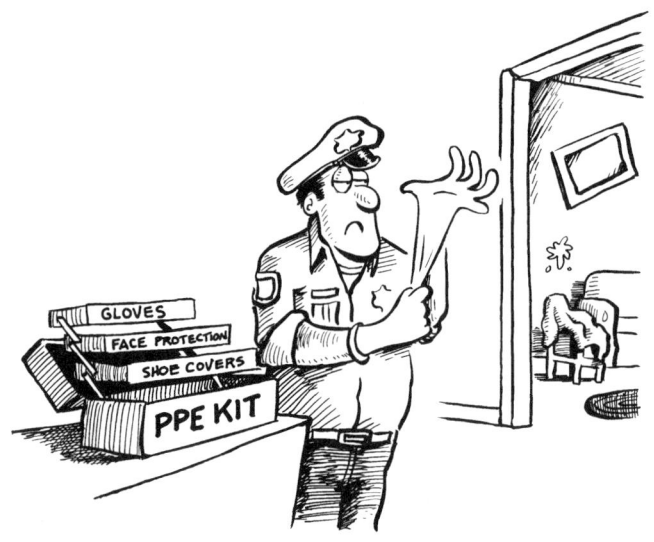

Wear PPE While Collecting Evidence

Minimize Splashing

Plan your activities to minimize or eliminate splashing and dripping of body fluids that might be infectious. Disease organisms can be spread if splashes and spatters of infected body fluids contact your eyes, nose, or mouth or areas of damaged skin. There's also a good chance that someone will touch body fluids accidentally and will spread them around the crime scene if splashing or spattering has occurred, thus increasing the risk of exposure. Make sure the containers you use for packaging won't spill or leak on the way back to the lab, or exposures could occur in this way too. Under **no** circumstances should you use a mouth pipette to collect wet body

> **Plan your activities to minimize splashing and dripping of body fluids.**

fluids. There's too much risk of getting infected fluid in your mouth with this procedure.

When drying material that is contaminated with potentially infectious body fluids, anticipate fluids dripping from this material, and take steps to minimize splashing. Post signs or warnings advising those entering the area that potentially infectious body fluids are present.

Use Tape, Not Staples

Items that are dripping wet with body fluids should be packaged in leakproof containers or in plastic bags before being transported to the lab, in order to avoid leaks of potentially infectious materials during transport. If there is little risk of leaking, items needed as evidence, such as clothing, bedding, and dried blood samples, can be wrapped in paper or packaged in paper bags for transportation, in accordance with accepted crime scene procedures. When sealing the bags, use tape rather than staples. Staples can tear gloves and cause puncture wounds. They also make holes in the collection bags, which can let contaminants seep out and can lead to cross contamination. Using tape will eliminate these risks.

> **Staples can tear gloves and let contaminants leak out of collection bags.**

Use Tweezers for Glass

Broken glass and other contaminated sharp items can easily cause cuts even if you're trying to be careful. Latex or vinyl gloves offer little protection in this situation. To be safe, never try to pick up glass with your bare hands or even with gloves on. Instead, use tweezers, prongs, or some other device, while being extremely careful not to destroy evidence. Place the items in a puncture resistant container with a tight fitting lid, not in a plastic bag. It's too easy for a bag to tear during handling, resulting in possible loss of evidence, injury to the handler, and exposure to a communicable disease.

For large items such as knives, axes, and machetes, carefully protect the sharp edge and the entire device, following standard evidence collection procedures. Think about the safety of personnel who will handle the item after you do, and take any additional precautions necessary to ensure that others will not be injured while handling the evidence.

Use Warning Labels

As you work, take time to label each evidence package clearly with a warning indicating that the contents might be infectious. Use either a written warning statement or a biohazard sticker on each bag or container. Such warnings should accompany evidence packages at all times so everyone handling the containers, including lab personnel, prosecutors, and defense lawyers, will be alerted to the hazards. To avoid having to remove potentially infectious evidence from its packaging in the courtroom, place items in transparent packaging once they've been properly dried, and affix appropriate identifying markings in a clearly visible location.[1]

> **Label evidence packages with warnings indicating the presence of potentially infectious materials.**

Handle Collection Tools Properly

As soon as you finish using each evidence collection tool, pack the instrument in a plastic bag that is clearly marked to indicate that the item is contaminated. Don't just lay collection tools down somewhere or toss them in your vehicle. Don't throw them in a public trash container either. Such actions can spread contaminants and can result in exposure if someone touches a contaminated surface or rummages through the trash bin. Take the bagged collection tools back to the station with you and then either dispose of them or decontaminate them according to your department's requirements.

Pack evidence collection tools in plastic bags after use.

© 1996 onGUARD, Inc.

Once you've collected the evidence you need, it's time to decontaminate yourself and your equipment.

> **OBJECTIVE:** Summarize the steps you should follow to decontaminate yourself and your equipment after collecting evidence.

Key Points

1. Properly **remove** and either **dispose of** or **decontaminate** all **personal protective equipment** in accordance with specific department regulations.

2. Follow departmental guidelines for **cleaning** your **clothing.**

3. **Wash** your **hands** and other **exposed skin** areas.

4. **Decontaminate** nondisposable items, such as **cameras, notebooks,** and **eyeglasses.**

Remove PPE

Personal protective equipment used during evidence collection may appear uncontaminated if no splashes or spatters of body fluids occurred. Remember, though, that dried body fluids are often hard to see, and disease organisms in body fluids are invisible to the naked eye. It's important that you use care as you remove PPE so you don't spread contaminants. Specifically, don't let the outer surfaces of gloves, protective eyewear, or body covering touch your skin or clothing as you take PPE off. You may want to practice putting on and removing PPE, especially gloves, several times until you can perform the procedure without contaminating yourself.

> **Remove PPE carefully so the outer surfaces don't touch your skin or clothing.**

As with the tools that you use for evidence collection, don't lay any used PPE down at the scene of the crime or dispose of it in a public trash container, since disease organisms can be spread in this way. In Odessa, Texas, three preschool children found a pair of bloody gloves outside an apartment where an intravenous drug user had died of an overdose. The gloves had apparently been left at the scene by emergency response personnel. The children tried to inflate the gloves with their mouths, since they had seen someone blow up a glove like a balloon in a hospital emergency room. A $2 million lawsuit was subsequently filed against the Ector County Sheriff's Department as a result of the incident, claiming that the parents of the children deserved compensation for their medical expenses and mental anguish while they waited to hear whether their children had been infected with HIV.[2]

To avoid a repeat of this type of situation in your own department, be sure to take all gloves and other PPE with you when you leave an emergency scene. Place used PPE in leakproof plastic bags marked with a biohazard symbol. Take the bags back to the police station, and then either dispose of the PPE or clean the items in accordance with department policy.

Remove and Clean Contaminated Clothing

While you're removing PPE, also remove any clothing that may have come in contact with blood or other body fluids, if practical. Place contaminated items in a leakproof plastic bag, as above. Follow departmental guidelines for cleaning your clothing once you return to the station.

Wash Hands and Skin

Perform handwashing at the emergency scene, if possible. Use a waterless hand cleaner if running water isn't available. Rewash your hands and any exposed skin areas as soon as you can, using soap and warm running water.

Frequent handwashing is one of the best ways to prevent the spread of communicable diseases. Either liquid or granular soap is recommended. Avoid using a bar of soap, if you can, or you'll end up washing yourself with the remnants of what the last person left behind. Soap dispensers can easily be mounted next to sinks. Using them will eliminate the risk of cross contamination.

> **Using a bar of soap means washing with the remnants of what the last person left behind.**

Decontaminate Nondisposable Items

Items such as cameras, notebooks, and prescription eyeglasses will need to be decontaminated if they were exposed to any body fluids at the crime scene. Even if these items were not splashed or spattered directly, if you happened to touch them while wearing contaminated gloves, you'll still need to decontaminate them. Follow your department's regulations and use common sense when cleaning such items. Pens and pencils are often more easily disposed of than disinfected.

> **Cameras, notebooks, and eyeglasses may need to be cleaned too.**

Summary

A "cold" crime scene is a controlled situation, but it isn't risk free when it comes to the possibility of transmission of a communicable disease. When investigating such a scene, wear gloves as minimum protection. Refrain from smoking, eating, and drinking while on-scene, and be careful not to put pencils or other objects in your mouth. Try not to touch your eyes, nose, or mouth if your hands might be contaminated.

When collecting evidence, follow accepted crime scene practices in everything you do. Wear a face mask, eye protection, and body covering in addition to gloves if there's a chance that spattering or splashing of body fluids might occur. Try to keep splashing to a minimum as you work. Pack wet body fluids in spillproof and leakproof containers. Seal plastic bags used for storing evidence with tape, not

© 1996 OnGUARD, Inc.

staples, to prevent accidental injury during handling of the containers. Use tweezers or some other device to pick up broken glass and other sharp fragments, and put the pieces in a puncture resistant container. Label all collection containers with appropriate warnings indicating the presence of potentially infectious materials. Pack tools used for evidence collection in plastic bags after use. Don't leave any tools at the scene of the crime. Instead, take them back to the station for either disposal or decontamination.

Carry out personal decontamination after completing the evidence collection process. This process involves removing personal protective equipment and contaminated clothing, either disposing of the items or cleaning them, and then washing your hands and exposed skin areas. You may also need to decontaminate nondisposable items such as cameras, notebooks, and eyeglasses after returning to the station.

References and Recommended Reading

1. Bigbee, P. D. (1987). Collecting and handling evidence infected with human disease-causing organisms. *FBI Law Enforcement Bulletin, 56*(7), p. 4.
2. Garza, M. A. (1992). Inside EMS. *Journal of Emergency Medical Services, 17*(9), p. 34.

SESSION 6
Bookings and Legal Issues

The need for infection control procedures doesn't end once a suspect has been arrested and evidence has been collected at the scene of a crime. Precautions are also needed during the booking process at the detention facility and during routine activities such as cleaning a holding cell. In this session, we'll outline appropriate procedures to use in these settings.

We'll also address some of the legal issues that law enforcement agencies face nowadays in trying to create a safe working environment for their employees. We touched on these in Session 1. Here we'll go into more detail about laws, court rulings, training requirements, confidentiality, and other matters.

> **Agencies face numerous legal issues related to communicable diseases.**

> **Scenario 6-1: Booking a Prisoner**
>
> *You're the booking officer in a prisoner intake area. The arresting officer has just brought in a prisoner who looks as though he's been in a fight. His hands and clothing are bloodied. He's also coughing, and you suspect he may have tuberculosis. He has already been searched thoroughly for weapons.*

> ***OBJECTIVE:** Identify precautions you should take when fingerprinting and searching a prisoner to guard against exposure to a communicable disease.*

Key Points

1. Wear *gloves.*

2. Have the *prisoner empty* his or her own *pockets.*

3. Wear a *face mask* and *protective eyewear* if the prisoner is *coughing.*

Wear Gloves

As we've already stressed many times, if there's a reasonable likelihood that you could touch blood or other body fluids and you have time to put on gloves first, do so. Booking a prisoner is a controlled situation, just like investigating a cold crime scene. For your own protection, take advantage of the chance to put on personal protective equipment before you get involved. In Scenario 6-1, the blood on the prisoner's hands and clothing should prompt you to get out your gloves without a moment's hesitation before you start the booking process.

Even if you can't see any blood on a subject, it's a good idea to wear gloves anyway, since other infected body fluids could be present. Wearing gloves while you perform fingerprinting will shield you from any blood or other body fluids a prisoner may have on his or her hands. Gloves will also protect you while you're conducting a search, as long as the gloves don't get punctured or torn. Remember to proceed slowly and cautiously during a search so you don't get poked or cut by hidden syringes, razor blades, or other sharp items. Gloves provide only limited protection against such objects.

> **Wear gloves while fingerprinting and searching a prisoner.**

It's often useful to ask subjects if they have any concealed sharp objects before you begin a search. You may also want to use an object such as a pen to detect hard items underneath clothing before you actually touch a person.

Change gloves every time you deal with a new prisoner. If you should get disease organisms on your gloves during a search, you could transfer the organisms to the next person you touch if you don't change gloves, which could create a liability issue for your department.

Have Prisoners Empty Pockets

In some situations, you may be able to eliminate the risk of getting cut or jabbed by a sharp object during a search by asking a prisoner to empty his or her own pockets, cuffs, socks, and shoes. Before you make such a request, though, evaluate the following:

> **Asking subjects to empty their own pockets can reduce the risk of cuts and needlesticks.**

- Is this a controlled environment?
- Has the suspect been thoroughly searched for weapons prior to arrival at the booking office?
- Is there a possibility that the suspect could destroy evidence while emptying his or her pockets?
- Is the suspect cooperative?

If any of these areas is questionable, it's best to empty pockets and other concealed areas yourself.

If you need to search a purse, carefully turn the purse upside down over a flat surface, such as a desk or table (if you're outdoors, use the hood of a car or the ground), and empty the contents that way rather than reaching inside.

© 1996 OnGUARD, Inc.

By not reaching into areas where you can't see what you're doing, you'll avoid unwanted contact with needles or other sharp objects. Make good use of every opportunity you get to reduce the risk of exposure to a communicable disease!

Wear Face/Eye Protection for Coughing

Coughing can spread airborne disease organisms, such as tuberculosis bacteria and measles viruses. One way to protect yourself from such organisms is to wear a face mask and protective eyewear if you need to be in close contact with someone who's coughing. An alternative is to put a mask on the subject, as long as the mask doesn't interfere with the person's ability to breathe. In Scenario 6-1, since the prisoner is coughing and you think he might have TB, you're wise either to put a mask and eye protection on yourself or to put a mask on the prisoner, or both, during the booking process.

© 1996 OnGUARD, Inc.

Scenario 6-2: Cleaning a Cell

You finish booking the prisoner described in Scenario 6-1 and put him in a holding cell. When you return a few minutes later, you find that he has vomited in the cell, contaminating both the walls and the floor.

OBJECTIVE: State the procedures you should follow in cleaning a cell so there will be minimal risk of exposure to a communicable disease.

Key Points

1. Wear **utility gloves, face protection, body covering,** and **shoe coverings.**

2. **Soak up body fluids, sweep** up loose dirt, **scrub** surfaces with soap and hot water, **apply bleach** solution, and **air dry.**

3. **Dispose of** or **decontaminate cleaning materials.**

4. **Decontaminate yourself.**

Wear PPE

Cleaning a cell is much like decontaminating a vehicle. You need full protection, including utility cleaning gloves, face and eye protection, body covering, and shoe coverings. Even if you're careful as you work, splashes and spatters are apt to occur. It's best to go into the situation armed with plenty of PPE.

> Cleaning a prison cell calls for full hand, face, and body protection.

Decontaminate Cell

Follow essentially the same steps for cleaning a cell as for cleaning a vehicle. In other words:

- Soak up wet body fluids with paper towels, rags, or other absorbent materials.

- **Carefully** sweep up loose dirt using a broom and dust pan. Be gentle here: if you sweep too vigorously, you could spatter potentially infectious materials onto the walls and furniture.

- Apply hot soapy water to any areas having visible contaminants. Then using a stiff brush, thoroughly scrub surfaces, paying special attention to corners and cracks. Mop up excess liquid when you're done.

- Apply a bleach solution to disinfect the cell. Start with the walls and then do the floor. Be sure to disinfect the entire cell, not just the areas that were visibly contaminated. As noted previously, bleach solutions should be

© 1996 OnGUARD, Inc.

made up fresh daily. Since there's little danger of damaging equipment or surfaces in a cell, a fairly strong bleach solution made by mixing one part bleach in 10 parts water (1:10 concentration) can be used, or you can use an EPA registered disinfectant.

- Allow the bleach solution to air dry. Don't try to rush the drying process by wiping the surfaces, or you'll remove the disinfectant.

Dispose of or Decontaminate Cleaning Materials

Materials such as paper towels or rags that were used to soak up body fluids should be disposed of in accordance with specific departmental guidelines. Leakproof plastic bags marked with a biohazard symbol are commonly used for such waste. Under no circumstances should you throw contaminated waste in an ordinary trash container, where it could contaminate someone handling the trash.

> **Never dispose of contaminated waste materials in ordinary trash containers.**

Soapy water should be disposed of in a mop sink or floor drain. Decontaminate brushes, mops, sponges, buckets, and other items used in the cleaning process by rinsing them with a fresh bleach solution and then air drying. Either dispose of or decontaminate your gloves, face and eye protection, body covering, and shoe coverings as your department specifies.

Decontaminate Yourself

Complete the cleaning process by decontaminating yourself. This means changing your clothes, if necessary, and then carefully washing your hands and any other skin areas that might have been splashed or spattered. If your eyes, nose, and/or mouth were splashed, rinse them repeatedly with water.

Clean your clothing as your department outlines. It's best not to wash your uniform at home or in a public laundry, because doing so can spread contaminants. A cleaning contract with a local cleaning company is usually the best way to handle contaminated laundry.

> **Personal decontamination is an essential part of the cleaning process.**

Any training program on infection control would be incomplete without a discussion of the current issues facing law enforcement agencies. Let's see what some of these concerns are.

> **OBJECTIVE: Summarize the major legal issues relating to infection control that law enforcement agencies need to address.**

Key Points

1. Police departments must provide **protection and services** to the public **without discrimination.**

2. Many employers are bound by **OSHA regulations** or follow **guidelines** published by **CDC.**

3. Employers are **not allowed** to **segregate, fire,** or **demote** an employee if the person becomes infected with a communicable disease.

4. **Confidentiality** of a person's disease status must be **balanced against** needs for **disclosure.**

5. The **Ryan White Act** sets forth procedures allowing officers to be **notified** if a hospitalized subject has a communicable disease.

6. **Documentation** of exposure incidents is essential for obtaining **workers' compensation benefits.**

7. Law enforcement agencies must provide **adequate training** to their employees regarding communicable diseases.

8. In **prisons,** hot issues include **mass screening** for HIV and **segregation** of inmates infected with HIV.

9. Agencies should **go beyond what's required** of them in protecting their employees.

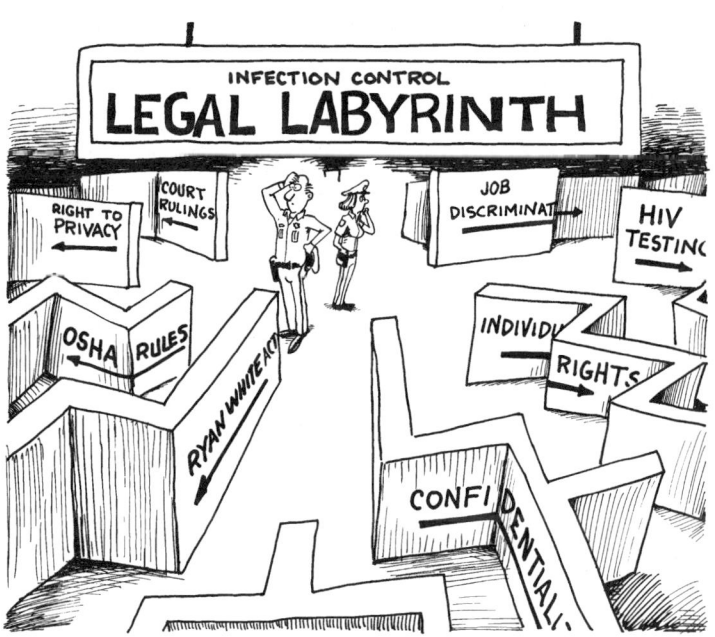

Learn Relevant Legal Issues

© 1996 OnGUARD, Inc.

No Discrimination

> **Fear of HIV doesn't free you from your obligation to perform your duties.**

The Constitution of the United States provides that American citizens are entitled to equal protection of the laws. Police officers, like other public servants and employees, may not discriminate and select the types of people they serve or the services they provide. Fear of HIV, for example, is not a justifiable reason to withhold police services, whether you're performing a search, handling evidence, making an arrest, or carrying out other duties.

OSHA and CDC

The Occupational Safety and Health Administration (OSHA) is a federal agency in the Department of Labor that is responsible for establishing requirements for protecting the lives and health of employees. Through the Occupational Safety and Health Act of 1970,[1] regulations have been enacted that are designed to protect private employees and to require employers to take steps to provide a safe working environment. As currently written, the law applies to all states, but it exempts federal and state employees. Some states have enacted laws that meet or exceed the federal OSHA requirements and have submitted a plan to OSHA for approval. These state plans protect both state and private employees. **Agencies should be sure what laws and/or policies they operate under.**

OSHA has recognized the need for required safeguards to protect workers against hazards related to infectious materials. OSHA enacted regulations known as the *Occupational Exposure to Bloodborne Pathogens Final Rule*, or

OSHA Final Rule,[2] which went into effect on March 6, 1992. These regulations create a standard in training and management of infection control matters. Although the OSHA Final Rule and CDC guidelines (discussed below) may not be legal mandates for some police agencies or jurisdictions, they were developed based on years of study, research, and public hearings, and they serve as **the** benchmark for protecting employee health and safety. Law enforcement agencies are well advised to adhere to their recommendations.

The goal of the OSHA Final Rule is to reduce the risk of occupational exposures to bloodborne diseases and to limit the impact of exposures that do occur. Important provisions of this Rule include the following:

- Employee positions that are at risk of exposure must be identified.

- Procedures for evaluating the circumstances surrounding an exposure incident must be outlined.

- Training must be provided regarding bloodborne pathogens, the ways bloodborne diseases are transmitted, and the obligations of employers if an exposure occurs. Retraining is to be done on a yearly basis.

- A written, comprehensive, exposure control plan must be established. This plan must address training, follow-up procedures for exposures, recordkeeping of medical reports, and a schedule for cleaning facilities and equipment that may be contaminated.

- Hepatitis B vaccinations must be made available to all employees who are at risk of contacting infected con-

> **The OSHA Final Rule outlines procedures that some employers must follow to reduce exposures to bloodborne diseases.**

taminated materials on the job. If an employee declines the vaccination series, this must be noted in writing.

- Employers must provide appropriate personal protective equipment, such as masks, protective eyewear, and gloves, at no cost to employees.
- Employers must provide medical follow-up in the event an exposure incident occurs, at no cost to employees.
- Employers must maintain training records and medical records.

> **CDC guidelines aren't laws, but they reflect appropriate and widely accepted standards.**

The Centers for Disease Control and Prevention (CDC) is a federal agency in the Department of Health and Human Services that conducts research and collects information about diseases and disease transmission. It also publishes guidelines that are widely accepted in the government and private sectors. One important document that CDC has published is entitled *Guidelines for Prevention of Transmission of Human Immunodeficiency Virus and Hepatitis B Virus to Health-Care and Public-Safety Workers.*[3] This document reflects the risk of exposure that public safety officers face and the preventive measures that are necessary to reduce employee exposures to HIV and hepatitis B.

Job Discrimination

The Rehabilitation Act of 1973 prohibits employers who receive federal funds from discriminating against employees who have handicaps but who are able to perform their job assignments. The law also requires employers to attempt to accommodate employees with handicaps, unless doing so causes undue hardship for the employer. According to a legal opinion issued by the Department of Justice in 1988, individuals who are infected with HIV are protected by the Rehabilitation Act, whether they show symptoms of the disease or not. In 1987, the United States Supreme Court ruled that a school teacher with tuberculosis was considered to have a handicap that was protected by this law. Therefore, she could not be terminated from her position solely because of her disease diagnosis. The court also ruled that consideration to offering her alternative employment should have been made by the employer.[4]

> **Employers are not allowed to discriminate against employees who have handicaps.**

A firefighter applicant argued the Rehabilitation Act when he had successfully completed all prerequisites to employment but wasn't allowed to fill the position. He was able to establish that although he had been offered the job, he wasn't allowed to work because he had informed the District of Columbia Fire Department that he was HIV positive. The firefighter didn't have any symptoms of HIV and was able to meet the physical requirements of the position. In addition, the District of Columbia could not establish that the applicant posed a "direct threat" to the health and safety of the public. A "direct threat" is defined as a significant risk that cannot be eliminated by a change in policies or practice, or with the assistance of aids or services. Factors considered in this determination include the type, duration, and severity of the risk and the probability of disease transmission.[5] Because HIV is not transmitted through casual contact, it was held that the firefighter did not pose a risk to the public. This firefighter was allowed to fill the position of firefighter, and he also recovered damages from the fire agency.

The Rehabilitation Act and the court cases that interpret it provide you with support if you become infected with a communicable disease. The law forbids segregation or discrimination against you if you are considered "handicapped" under the law. You are entitled to remain employed, so long as you're able to fulfill your job responsibilities, just like any other employee. You may not be terminated solely because of your disease status. In all situations, you should be given the same degree of respect, fairness, and dignity as any other person.

> **Employees may not be terminated solely because of their disease status.**

In 1990, a federal law entitled the Americans with Disabilities Act, or ADA,[6] was enacted. This law goes beyond the Rehabilitation Act and requires essentially all private employers, state and local governmental employers, and labor unions to refrain from discrimination in employment practices. The law prohibits employment discrimination against "qualified individuals with disabilities," which includes persons with HIV infection.

Confidentiality

Medical information about a person is usually considered private, and generally there is an expectation that this information will not be disclosed. However, there is also an overwhelming public interest in preventing the spread of communicable diseases, which has complicated the interest of privacy. The rights of individuals who are suspected or known to be infected with a communicable disease are balanced against the valid needs of the public, coworkers, victims, and suspects. Some states have enacted specific statutes prohibiting disclosure of HIV information and imposing criminal or civil sanctions.

The interest in confidentiality constantly faces competing disclosure questions. As a peace officer, you should be informed about when disclosures are allowed or prohibited. State statutes are continually being enacted and interpreted by the courts. These laws impact the testing of individuals for communicable diseases, disclosure of test results, and other uses of this information. For example, in many states, only medical care providers treating an HIV infected inmate are authorized to know the communicable disease status of an inmate.[7] One state allows probation officers to inform local law enforcement of a probationer's HIV positive status if an arrest of the person is to be made and the person has a history of assault on a police officer.[8] Because there are many, many different statutory provisions, you should take time to learn your state's specific laws and regulations about this sensitive area.

> **The interest in confidentiality constantly faces competing disclosure questions.**

Confidentiality and disclosure can also be at odds regarding the results of tests done for communicable diseases, particularly in the context of victims of crimes in which HIV could be transmitted. At issue are the competing interests of the victim and the defendant. It may be important for a law enforcement officer to know a defendant's HIV status to determine what criminal charges can be filed. This is especially true in states, such as Georgia, where conduct may constitute an "AIDS transmitting crime."[9] In some states, testing and disclosure of test results are not allowed until after the defendant is convicted of criminal conduct.

There have been several court cases involving security or peace officers who were bitten by a person, and the officers wanted the assailants to be tested for HIV. In

© 1996 OnGUARD, Inc.

California, where a deputy sought involuntary testing of a woman who bit him, the court authorized the test.[10] California's statute allows testing if there is probable cause to believe that "a possible transfer of blood" has occurred between a defendant and a peace officer.[11] In Florida, a statute allows involuntary testing if a law enforcement officer sustains an injury on the job "such as to result in the transmission" of a communicable disease.[12]

Again, because of the range of state laws, it's important that you study your state's regulations before you say anything to anyone about a person's communicable disease status or request communicable disease testing. Additional suggestions for keeping information confidential are listed in Figure 6-1.

Recommendations for Preserving Confidentiality

- ❖ Don't discuss encounters or the names of subjects publicly.
- ❖ Don't discuss previous subjects or incidents in the presence of subjects.
- ❖ Minimize radio transmissions that reveal personal information.
- ❖ Don't leave reports in public places, such as on counters.
- ❖ Don't reveal an individual's communicable disease status to anyone who isn't authorized to know. This includes sharing information with fellow officers; other criminal justice agencies; public health departments; and spouses, other family members, sexual partners, and employers of infected individuals.
- ❖ Maintain the confidentiality of the results of any tests, such as HIV antibody tests and tuberculosis tests.

Figure 6-1

Ryan White Act

Documentation of exposure incidents becomes important under the Ryan White Act (technically, the Ryan White Comprehensive AIDS Resources Emergency Act of 1990[13]). This law provides a notification process for emergency responders who may have had an exposure incident with a victim of an emergency. If the victim is transported to a hospital, the peace officer can request, in writing, that the hospital evaluate whether or not an exposure to a communicable disease occurred. The notification to the emergency responder must be accomplished within 48 hours after the request was made.

> The Ryan White Act allows hospitals to release a patient's communicable disease status if an exposure occurred.

Under proposed rules for the implementation of the Ryan White Act, the term "emergency response employees" includes law enforcement officers, and the "patient" is a "victim of an emergency who has been aided" by an emergency responder and transported to a medical facility.[14] When the provisions of the Ryan White Act are in effect, they should enable law enforcement personnel throughout the country to gain a little peace of mind about whether or not an exposure to an infected patient occurred. Obviously, the documentation of the incident will be critical to benefiting from the law, since the hospital evaluates the request before it determines if the possible source patient's records need to be reviewed.

© 1996 OnGUARD, Inc.

Workers' Compensation

As a peace officer, you have the right to confidentiality in accordance with state laws. If you're exposed to a communicable disease during your work, you may be entitled to seek workers' compensation benefits. The documentation about your injury, your medical records, and follow-up reports relating to your exposure should be kept confidential at your place of employment. If you are reassigned to a different work position because of a medical condition, the reassignment should also be maintained confidentially. Disclosures should be limited to those who have a valid need to know this information.

> **Documentation about any exposure incident is critical to obtaining compensation benefits.**

Documentation about any exposure incident is critical to obtaining compensation benefits. It's important to document in detail the facts of the incident—how you were exposed (e.g., blood to blood contact), whether you were wearing personal protective equipment and its integrity, and what cleaning efforts you made immediately after the incident. Only if there is sufficient information to establish that the exposure occurred while you were performing your job will you be able to get the benefits you need.

Training

Every law enforcement department should receive training about communicable diseases, including when disclosures about a person's disease status should and should not be made. These principles were specifically addressed in a New Jersey case, in which the family of a man who was infected with HIV sued the municipal police department. The man's HIV status was disclosed by a police officer to members of the public who had not had any contact with the man and therefore had no need to know the disease status, which violated the family's right to privacy. In addition, the police department failed to provide its officers with any training about disease transmission, despite knowledge that other law enforcement departments had been trained about infection precautions and despite the public's misperceptions about HIV transmission. This failure to provide training, according to *Doe v. Borough of Barrington*, constituted deliberate indifference to the privacy rights of the family.[15]

In 1989, the United States Supreme Court ruled that a municipality's failure to train can reflect a deliberate or conscious choice of indifference to the rights of the citizens it serves. This case, *City of Canton v. Harris*,[16] stands for the proposition that ignorance among law enforcement departments is not tolerated where citizens' civil rights are involved.

> **Ignorance among law enforcement departments is not tolerated where citizens' civil rights are involved.**

Training is also essential in correctional facilities. Any training about HIV infection should emphasize that the disease is **not** spread by casual contact. Clear explanations should be provided about how guards and inmates can avoid becoming infected by any communicable disease. New inmates as well as guard personnel should be trained, because "fears resurface when education and training lapse."[17] Information helps allay these fears and allows guards to do their job with less stress and risk.

Other Prison Issues

In correctional facilities in some states, HIV screening is done to identify if new inmates are HIV positive. The problem with this approach is that a single, isolated test does not prevent disease transmission. A test does not assure the correctional staff that inmates will not become positive for HIV or any other disease. Consequently, the test is of little help to guards. In addition, the need for a correctional officer to know the HIV status of all inmates is questionable. If an inmate's disease status is known, the guard must still honor the person's privacy interest, must still practice safe infection control techniques, and must still refrain from disclosing this medical information except in accordance with state and federal laws.

> Mass screening for HIV and segregation of inmates infected with HIV are important issues in some prisons.

Inmates who are HIV positive are segregated in several states. However, it is questionable whether this practice prevents disease transmission. Since HIV is not transmitted through casual contact, it is reasonable that segregation may only be warranted where an infected inmate's actions put others at risk for infection.[18] Disease transmission has not been successfully prevented simply by isolating inmates who were screened at a particular point in time. Nonetheless, isolation of HIV infected inmates has been allowed by the courts. Inmates have challenged segregation, claiming unequal protection of the laws, but they have had little success.[19] The bottom line is that training is still essential in custodial facilities.

A Step Further

For the war against communicable diseases to be effective, law enforcement agencies need to go beyond the basic requirements of the law and take the next step in protecting their employees. Three areas should be addressed:

- Departments should provide separate facilities for personal decontamination and for cleaning and disposal of contaminated materials. The use of a bathroom or kitchen sink to clean contaminated items or to perform personal decontamination leaves a lot of room for cross contamination. So does disposing of contaminated items with regular trash. A separate decontamination area and designated containers for contaminated waste are recommended.

  > **Agencies need to go beyond the basic requirements of the law.**

- Patrol cars, booking areas, and detention facilities should all be stocked with adequate supplies of personal protective equipment and cleaning materials. Recommended supplies are listed in Figure 6-2. If you use any of the materials, get in the habit of replacing them as soon as possible. Don't expect someone else to do it. It should be every person's responsibility to maintain a complete inventory of supplies.

Recommended Infection Control Supplies

- ✓ Disposable latex or vinyl gloves in various sizes
- ✓ Leather gloves
- ✓ Protective eyewear
- ✓ Face masks
- ✓ Resuscitation equipment with a one way valve
- ✓ Clean coveralls or other body protection in appropriate sizes
- ✓ Disposable shoe coverings
- ✓ Puncture resistant containers for sharp objects
- ✓ Leakproof plastic bags imprinted with the biohazard symbol
- ✓ Tape for sealing bags
- ✓ Bags for normal waste
- ✓ Waterless handwashing cleanser
- ✓ Waterproof bandages
- ✓ Absorbent cleaning materials for spills
- ✓ "Isolation Area–Do Not Enter" signs

Figure 6-2

- Adequate department policies should be developed and communicated to all personnel. These policies should cover all areas of infection control, including the following:
  - ✓ training requirements
  - ✓ vaccinations
  - ✓ personal protective equipment
  - ✓ personal decontamination
  - ✓ decontamination of equipment and clothing
  - ✓ handling of sharp objects
  - ✓ disposal of contaminated items
  - ✓ what to do if an exposure occurs
  - ✓ confidentiality

Make sure the policies are communicated clearly to everyone in the department, or they won't be effective. Yearly refresher sessions are recommended.

Summary

Infection control procedures are needed in controlled situations such as booking a prisoner and cleaning a holding cell, just as they are in other types of incidents. When booking a prisoner, always wear gloves, and have prisoners empty their own pockets, if possible. When searching a purse, empty the contents over a flat surface instead of reaching inside. If the subject is coughing, put on a face mask to protect yourself from airborne diseases.

Cleaning a holding cell calls for full hand, face, and body protection to guard against splashes. Scrub surfaces with soap and water, and then disinfect with a bleach solution. Decontaminate the cleaning materials after the job is finished, and then perform thorough personal decontamination.

There are several important legal issues relating to infection control that affect all departments providing police services. State and federal laws prohibit discrimination in the provision of protection or services. In addition, many departments are subject to regulations and guidelines set forth in the OSHA Final Rule and in documents produced by the Centers for Disease Control and Prevention. You need to be aware of local regulations on confidentiality and disclosure of communicable disease status. If you experience an exposure, the Ryan White Act may help you obtain information on the communicable disease status of the source patient. Documentation of exposure incidents is critical in obtaining compensation benefits. If you become infected on the job, your employer is not allowed to fire you solely because of your disease status.

Agencies have a responsibility to provide adequate training to their employees regarding infection control. Correctional facilities also need to train inmates about how to prevent the spread of communicable diseases. Other issues that may need to be addressed in prisons are mass screening for HIV and segregation of infected inmates.

Agencies are urged to go beyond the basic requirements of the law when it comes to creating a safe work environment for their employees. Recommended actions include providing separate facilities for decontamination, providing adequate supplies of personal protective equipment, and implementing infection control policies throughout the department.

References and Recommended Reading

1. Public Law 91-596, 28 U.S.C.A. Section 651 et seq.
2. 29 CFR Part 1910.1030.
3. Centers for Disease Control. (1989, February). *Guidelines for prevention of transmission of human immunodeficiency virus and hepatitis B virus to health-care and public-safety workers* (DHHS Publication No. 89-107). Washington, DC: U.S. Government Printing Office.
4. *School Board of Nassau County v. Arline*, 480 U.S. 273 (1987).
5. 29 U.S.C. Section 706(8)(D) and *School Board of Nassau County v. Arline*.
6. Public Law 101-336.

© 1996 OnGUARD, Inc.

7. WIS. STATE ANN., Section 146.025(5)(a)(13) (West 1989).
8. CAL. PENAL LAW, Section 2782(1)(m) (McKinney Supp. 1990).
9. GA. CODE ANN., Section 15-11-35.1(d) (Supp. 1990).
10. *Johnetta J. v. Municipal Court*, 267 Cal. Rptr. 666 (Cal. App. 1 Dist. 1990).
11. CAL. HEALTH & SAFETY CODE, Section 199.97 (West 1989).
12. FLA. STATUTE, Section 796.08(7)(a) (Supp. 1990).
13. Public Law 101-381.
14. Centers for Disease Control and Prevention (1992, November 20). Proposed implementation of provisions of the Ryan White CARE Act regarding emergency response employees. *Federal Register, 57*(225), p. 54795.
15. *Doe v. Borough of Barrington*, 729 F. Supp. 376 (Dist. N.J., 1990).
16. *City of Canton v. Harris*, 489 U.S. 378, 109 S. Ct. 1197, 103 L. Ed. 2d 412 (1989).
17. Clark, M. E. (1990). AIDS prevention: Legislative options. *American Journal of Law and Medicine, 16*(1-2), p. 146.
18. Clark, M. E. (1990). AIDS prevention: Legislative options. *American Journal of Law and Medicine, 16*(1-2), p. 147.
19. *Cordero v. Coughlin*, 607 F. Supp. 9 (D.C.N.Y., 1984).

Notes

Appendix

Exposure Control Guidelines fo

Disease	Possible Mode of Transmission	Relative Risk for Police Officers
Chicken Pox	■ Breathing airborne droplets produced when an infected person coughs or sneezes. ■ Contact of fluid from moist blisters or with the mucous membranes of the eyes, nose, or mouth.	■ None, if you've ha chicken pox before. ■ Significant, if yo haven't had chicke pox.
Common Cold	■ Breathing airborne droplets produced when an infected person coughs or sneezes. ■ Contact of respiratory secretions with the mucous membranes of the eyes, nose, or mouth.	Unknown—Probab significant if cold is in th early stages.
Diarrhea	Eating or drinking food or water contaminated with the feces of an infected person.	Unknown—Probab low, providing you wa your hands after conta with feces.
Diphtheria	Breathing airborne droplets produced when an infected person coughs or sneezes.	Low.

© 1996 OnGUARD, Inc.

ommon Communicable Diseases

Recommended Precautions	Exposure Follow-Up
If you've had chicken pox, you n't get it again, so contact with an ected person isn't a problem. If you haven't had chicken pox, try avoid contact with infected people. If you haven't had chicken pox and u need to deal with infected indi- luals, use appropriate BSI tech- ues for airborne diseases, i.e., ar a face mask, if possible. Put a face mask on infected adults. n't try to put a mask on a child. Wash your hands thoroughly after ching moist blisters. Use an airway device with a one y valve when performing resusci- ion on an infected person.	Contact a physician within 96 hours of exposure.
Don't touch your eyes, nose, or uth while dealing with an infected rson. Use appropriate BSI techniques airborne diseases. Wash your hands thoroughly after ntact with an infected person.	Contact a physician if symptoms develop and persist.
Wear gloves for direct contact with es. Wash your hands thoroughly after ntact with feces.	Contact a physician if symptoms develop and persist.
Use appropriate BSI techniques airborne diseases. Put a face mask on infected adults. n't try to put a mask on a child.	Contact a physician.

© 1996 OnGUARD, Inc.

Exposure Control Guidelines fo[r]

Disease	Possible Mode of Transmission	Relative Risk for Police Officers
Hepatitis A	Eating or drinking food or water contaminated with the feces or urine of an infected person.	Low.
Hepatitis B	■ Needlestick by a needle contaminated with infected blood. ■ Contact of infected blood or other infected body fluid with an open wound or damaged skin. ■ Contact of infected blood or other infected body fluid with the mucous membranes of the eyes, nose, or mouth.	Significant, if you hav[e] not had a hepatitis vaccination or if yo[u] don't get follow-up trea[t]ment after an exposur[e].
Hepatitis C	■ Needlestick by a needle contaminated with infected blood. ■ Contact of infected blood or other infected body fluid with an open wound or damaged skin. ■ Contact of infected blood or other infected body fluid with the mucous membranes of the eyes, nose, or mouth.	Unknown.
Hepatitis D	■ Needlestick by a needle contaminated with infected blood. ■ Contact of infected blood or other infected body fluid with an open wound or damaged skin. ■ Contact of infected blood or other infected body fluid with the mucous membranes of the eyes, nose, or mouth.	■ High, if you're cu[r]rently infected wit[h] hepatitis B. ■ None, if you don[']t have hepatitis B.
Hepatitis E	Eating or drinking food or water contaminated with the feces of an infected person.	Unknown.

© 1996 OnGUARD, Inc.

ommon Communicable Diseases

Recommended Precautions	Exposure Follow-Up
Avoid potentially contaminated ɔd or water. Wear gloves for direct contact with ɔes or urine. Wash your hands thoroughly after ntact with feces or urine.	Contact communicable disease personnel at your agency or local hospital.
ɪe appropriate BSI techniques for ɔodborne diseases.	■ Scrub exposed area with soap and water. ■ Contact communicable disease personnel at your agency or local hospital. ■ Follow appropriate procedures depending on your hepatitis B vaccine status.
ɪe appropriate BSI techniques for ɔodborne diseases.	■ Scrub exposed area with soap and water. ■ Contact communicable disease personnel at your agency or local hospital.
ɪe appropriate BSI techniques for ɔodborne diseases.	■ Scrub exposed area with soap and water. ■ Contact communicable disease personnel at your agency or local hospital.
Avoid potentially contaminated ɔd or water. Wear gloves for direct contact with ɔes. Wash your hands thoroughly after ntact with feces.	Contact communicable disease personnel at your agency or local hospital.

© 1996 OnGUARD, Inc.

Exposure Control Guidelines fo[r]

Disease	Possible Mode of Transmission	Relative Risk for Police Officer[s]
Herpes Simplex (Oral or Finger Infection)	■ Contact of fluid from moist blisters with the mucous membranes of the eyes, nose, or mouth. ■ Frequent contact of saliva from infected persons with broken skin, particularly on the fingers.	Unknown—Significan[t] blisters are presen[t] however, most peop[le] have antibodies.
Herpes Zoster (Shingles)	Contact of fluid from moist blisters with the mucous membranes of the eyes, nose, or mouth.	Moderate—If you hav[e] not had chicken po[x] you may get chicke[n] pox from someone w[ith] shingles (the disease[s] are caused by the sam[e] virus).
HIV/AIDS	■ Needlestick by a needle contaminated with infected blood. ■ Contact of infected blood with an open wound or with damaged skin. ■ Contact of infected blood with the mucous membranes of the eyes, nose, or mouth.	Low.
Influenza	Breathing airborne droplets produced when an infected person coughs or sneezes.	Unknown—Probab[ly] significant during f[lu] epidemics.
Lice	Close head to head contact or body contact.	High.

© 1996 OnGUARD, Inc.

Common Communicable Diseases

Recommended Precautions	Exposure Follow-Up
Wear gloves for contact with moist blisters or saliva. Wash your hands thoroughly after contact with saliva from an infected person.	Contact a physician if symptoms develop.
Shingles isn't a problem if you've had chicken pox. If you haven't had chicken pox, wash your hands thoroughly after contact with moist blisters.	Contact a physician if you haven't had chicken pox.
Use appropriate BSI techniques for bloodborne diseases.	■ Scrub exposed area with soap and water. ■ Contact communicable disease personnel at your agency or local hospital.
Use appropriate BSI techniques for airborne diseases. Put a mask on infected persons. Get an influenza vaccine.	Contact a physician if symptoms develop and persist.
Wash your hands thoroughly after contact with infested persons. Avoid head to head contact or body contact if lice are present.	■ Watch for lice eggs (nits) on hair shafts. ■ Contact a physician if significant exposure occurred.

© 1996 OnGUARD, Inc.

Exposure Control Guidelines fo[r]

Disease	Possible Mode of Transmission	Relative Risk for Police Officers
Measles	■ Breathing airborne droplets produced when an infected person coughs or sneezes. Be aware that measles is highly contagious. ■ Contact of nasal and throat secretions from an infected person with the mucous membranes of the eyes, nose, or mouth.	Unknown—Probab[ly] significant; howeve[r] most people have ant[i]bodies.
Meningitis (Bacterial)	■ Breathing airborne droplets produced when an infected person coughs or sneezes. ■ Contact with nasal and throat secretions from an infected person.	Unknown—Probabl[y] low.
Mumps	■ Breathing airborne droplets produced when an infected person coughs or sneezes. ■ Contact of saliva from an infected person with the mucous membranes of the eyes, nose, or mouth.	Unknown.
Rubella (German Measles)	■ Breathing airborne droplets produced when an infected person coughs or sneezes. ■ Contact of nasal and throat secretions from an infected person with the mucous membranes of the eyes, nose, or mouth.	Unknown—Susceptibl[e] persons are at i[n]creased risk.

© 1996 OnGUARD, Inc.

Common Communicable Diseases

Recommended Precautions	Exposure Follow-Up
Get a measles vaccine. If you've never had measles or a measles vaccine, avoid contact with infected persons. Use appropriate BSI techniques for airborne diseases.	■ Check your measles immunity. If you've had the disease, you're immune and you can't get measles again. If you haven't had measles but have been vaccinated, you should be immune. However, if you were born after 1957, you may need to be revaccinated; check with your public health department. ■ Notify your public health department of the exposure.
Use appropriate BSI techniques for airborne diseases.	Contact a physician within 24 hours of exposure to get preventive medication.
If you've never had mumps before, get a mumps vaccine and avoid contact with infected persons. Use appropriate BSI techniques for airborne diseases.	Contact a physician if symptoms develop.
Get a rubella vaccine. Use appropriate BSI techniques for airborne diseases.	■ If you've never had rubella, avoid contact with other susceptible persons. ■ If you're pregnant and aren't immune to rubella, contact your obstetrician. Rubella can cause serious birth defects in babies whose mothers contract the disease during the first three months of pregnancy.

© 1996 OnGUARD, Inc.

Exposure Control Guidelines fo[r]

Disease	Possible Mode of Transmission	Relative Risk for Police Officers
Scabies	Close body contact with an infested person.	Unknown—High if yo[u] have direct contact wit[h] an infested person.
Tuberculosis	Breathing airborne droplets produced when an infected person coughs or sneezes.	Unknown—Depends o[n] the level of the person'[s] infectivity, contact time[,] and ventilation.
Whooping Cough	Breathing airborne droplets produced when an infected person coughs or sneezes.	Unknown—Usually n[ot] a risk for adults.

© 1996 OnGUARD, Inc.